Pandemics: A Very Short Introduction

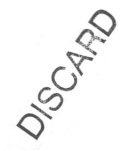

VERY SHORT INTRODUCTIONS are for anyone wanting a stimulating and accessible way into a new subject. They are written by experts, and have been translated into more than 40 different languages.

The series began in 1995, and now covers a wide variety of topics in every discipline. The VSI library now contains over 450 volumes—a Very Short Introduction to everything from Indian philosophy to psychology and American history and relativity—and continues to grow in every subject area.

Very Short Introductions available now:

Available soon:

For more information visit our website

www.oup.com/vsi/

Christian W. McMillen

PANDEMICS

A Very Short Introduction

OXFORD
UNIVERSITY PRESS

OXFORD

UNIVERSITY PRESS

Oxford University Press is a department of the University of Oxford.
It furthers the University's objective of excellence in research, scholarship,
and education by publishing worldwide. Oxford is a registered trade mark of
Oxford University Press in the UK and certain other countries.

Published in the United States of America by Oxford University Press
198 Madison Avenue, New York, NY 10016, United States of America.

© Oxford University Press 2016

Library of Congress Cataloging-in-Publication Data
Names: McMillen, Christian W., 1969- author.
Title: Pandemics : a very short introduction / Christian W. McMillen.
Description: New York, NY : Oxford University Press, [2016] | Series:
Very short introductions | Includes bibliographical references and index.
Identifiers: LCCN 2016028234| ISBN 9780199340071 (paperback) |
ISBN 9780199340088 (ebook updf) | ISBN 9780199340095 (ebook epub) |
ISBN 9780190625214 (online resource)
Subjects: LCSH: Epidemics—History. | BISAC: MEDICAL / History.
Classification: LCC RA649 .M373 2016 | DDC 614.4—dc23 LC record
available at https://lccn.loc.gov/2016028234

1 3 5 7 9 8 6 4 2

Printed in Great Britain
by Ashford Colour Press Ltd., Gosport, Hants.
on acid-free paper

For Olin, Maya, and Stephanie

Contents

List of illustrations

Acknowledgments

Several years ago Nancy Toff at Oxford and I met and discussed a variety of potential projects. I was then in the thick of working on a book on tuberculosis. Writing that book got me interested in epidemics more broadly. Nancy discovered, much to our mutual surprise, that there was no Very Short Introduction on either epidemics or pandemics. Maybe I could write such a book? With Nancy's help I did. Thanks, Nancy. Elda Granata at Oxford has been unflagging in her willingness to answer innumerable questions. She has made the process a pleasure. I am grateful to the students in my course Epidemics, Pandemics, and History for allowing me, without them knowing it, to test this material out on them. This book is based on the hard work of the many historians dedicated to making disease central to human history. My thanks to them. Finally, my wife, Stephanie, and our children, Maya and Olin, deserve, as always, my greatest thanks.

Introduction

This book will introduce readers to the rich history of pandemic and epidemic disease and suggest that much of the way we confront such things now has been shaped by the past. This is an unremarkable statement but an important point. For very often history is forgotten or rediscovered only when we confront contemporary epidemics and pandemics, and thus patterns from the past are repeated thoughtlessly.

What are pandemics and epidemics? An epidemic is generally considered to be an unexpected, widespread rise in disease incidence at a given time. A pandemic is best thought of as a very large epidemic. Ebola in 2014 was by any measure an epidemic—perhaps even a pandemic. The influenza that killed fifty million people around the world in 1918 was a pandemic.

A common way to think about epidemics and pandemics is as events. They come and they go. But if we think about them this way, can we call HIV/AIDS a pandemic? Or tuberculosis? What about malaria? Pandemics can be either discrete events or what I would like to call persistent pandemics. Tuberculosis, malaria, and HIV/AIDS, which affect enormous swaths of the globe and kill millions and millions each year, are persistent pandemics.

In the wake of the 2009 H1N1 influenza pandemic, controversy emerged over the definition of pandemics used by the World Health Organization (WHO) and others. In response, several infectious disease specialists at the National Institute of Allergy and Infectious Diseases at the National Institutes of Health (NIH) came up with a broad framework that can work to help define what a pandemic is and has been. They suggested that it must meet eight criteria: wide geographic extension, disease movement, high attack rates and explosiveness, minimal population immunity, novelty, infectiousness, contagiousness, and severity. It might seem that TB, HIV/AIDS, and malaria are not novel. But their profiles change—TB gets worse in one area, then better in another; XDR-TB emerges—and they become novel again. Each particular historical context is novel. Malaria took on a new identity in the 1950s when the WHO attempted to eradicate it; it took on another in the 1970s and 1980s as the World Bank became the major player in global health. Likewise with HIV/AIDS; its identity has changed so much over time that it has taken on multiple novel identities, each one historically contingent: a death sentence, a chronic and manageable infection, a gay disease, a heterosexual disease.

There are a number of themes and topics that link the history of epidemics and pandemics. The identities of each disease underwent significant change as a result of the late-nineteenth-century laboratory revolution—a revolution that ushered in the age of modern medicine in which we now live. What began with Louis Pasteur in France and culminated with the work of Robert Koch in Germany meant that diseases once explained in myriad ways were forever thereafter explained by one. The consequences of this change cannot be overstated. The discovery of bacteria as the cause of diseases such as tuberculosis meant that centuries-old explanations for disease etiology vanished. For the first time medical science actually knew what caused a given disease. Diseases might actually be able to be cured. The discovery of the tubercle bacillus and the bacteria that caused plague allowed medicine to develop effective therapies, as well as understand how to prevent infections. But the laboratory revolution also cultivated an undue amount of confidence in the power of biomedicine to rid the world of infectious diseases and fostered the belief that the way to do so was far more dependent on attacking germs than on attacking the social conditions that gave rise to disease in the first place.

This points to another pair of themes: the relationship between poverty and disease and the geography of epidemics and pandemics. All of the diseases discussed in this book, while able to be controlled (to varying degrees) by modern medicine, are affected by social conditions. That is, there is a reason cholera disappeared from the United States more than a century ago but is still present in much of the developing world, or that HIV/AIDS disproportionately effects sub-Saharan Africa, or that plague was worse among the poor than the rich during Marseilles's 1720 epidemic. Some places have been able to transcend the conditions that allow infectious diseases to flourish, while others have not.

These days most places with persistent pandemics are in what has come to be called the global south. The burden of epidemic disease has shifted: tuberculosis, once Europe's leading cause of death, has not disappeared from the earth; it has simply moved. TB declined in the West long before any effective therapy or preventive agent existed; it did so because of public health interventions such as isolation and a generally improved quality of life. TB has increased dramatically in the developing world even after the discovery of antibiotics—one of modern biomedicine's triumphs—that actually kill it and cure the patient. It has done so because of conditions that allow it to thrive: unequal access to drugs, crowded living conditions, high rates of infection, and comorbidities like HIV/AIDS, among other things. TB declined in one part of the world without the aid of biomedical interventions and increased in another part of the planet despite them.

None of this means that drugs and medical research are not essential for the control of epidemics. They are, of course.

Antiretroviral therapy, an extraordinary discovery by any measure, has been essential in the fight against HIV/AIDS. Yet access has been uneven, and infection rates are rising in some countries. Since its discovery in the 1960s, oral rehydration therapy for cholera has been lifesaving. But it does nothing to address the reasons why millions of people in the global south are drinking water contaminated by human feces. The very simple point is that there is a relationship between disease and social conditions, conditions that do not exist everywhere and that will not be alleviated with biomedicine.

Fear and dread characterize epidemics. Cholera caused considerable panic in the nineteenth century; those with HIV/AIDS inspired fear and discrimination in places like the United States in the recent past—and into the present. There is still considerable stigma attached to the disease. Plague prompted anti-Jewish pogroms in the fourteenth century. In our own time, the climate of fear in the United States during the 2014 Ebola pandemic was out of proportion to the actual risk. Yet influenza, which has the capacity to kill untold numbers (the 1918 pandemic killed at least fifty million people in less than a year), seems rarely to occasion much concern. Fearing some diseases and not others is often wrapped up in how a given disease manifests—cholera is a thoroughly unpleasant disease, the symptoms of which are dramatic and, to most sensibilities, disgusting—or how it is caused: HIV is tangled up in the complexities of human sexuality; many have perceived its causes to be rooted in social deviance, including intravenous drug use. A disease's place of origin can have an effect on whether it is feared or not. Malaria is now firmly a tropical disease in the developing world. When it appears occasionally in the developed north, it arrives as a frightening and exotic invader.

The question of susceptibility—who gets a disease and why—is important. In early America, colonists considered Indians to be virgin soil for smallpox and other Old World diseases. In the early decades of the twentieth century, black South Africans and others were thought to be racially susceptible to TB, while whites could fight infection. That Africans were less susceptible to malaria than colonists led, in part, to their importation as slaves to the New World in the seventeenth and eighteenth centuries. For hundreds of years, until the bacteriological revolution, many debated whether or not diseases were contagious or brought on by miasma—the bad air caused by rotting animal and vegetable matter. The plague was often considered to be a punishment for sin. Each of these explanations changed.

All of these diseases, save smallpox, are still with us. Only plague, which does still occur—there was an epidemic in India in the 1990s, and it has regular outbreaks in Madagascar—has diminished in scope and ferocity. And new diseases are surely on the horizon. Thus, while much of this book is historical, it is not solely about history.

The connection between epidemics and pandemics and the growth of the modern state is clear. As early as the fifteenth century, in response to the plague, Italian city states formed state-sponsored boards of health. The cholera pandemics of the nineteenth century led to nationwide efforts at quarantine—efforts that could only be carried off by a central state. Measures such as compulsory vaccination also demonstrate this connection.

Epidemics and pandemics cannot occur without a dense and mobile population. None of these diseases emerged in pandemic form until humans had settled down to farm and begun trading with one another. Infectious diseases need to be transmitted from host to host to survive; that host must be susceptible. Smallpox remained such a killer among American Indians because it was able, over centuries, to find non-immune populations; once those populations diminished, the disease naturally declined. Trade and travel were well developed by the fourteenth century; the plague took advantage of this. TB exploded only when conditions allowed it: the densely packed cities and workplaces of industrializing Europe in the eighteenth century. AIDS has relied on human mobility to move around the globe. When pandemic influenza spread around most of the planet in a matter of months in 1918, it could only have done so because of the newly built transportation and trade networks and the heightened mobility brought on by World War I. Human, animal, and insect movement are critical in the spread of epidemics and pandemics.

Finally, people—eyewitnesses, novelists, poets, memoirists, government bureaucrats, journalists, historians, anthropologists, epidemiologists, kings, queens, and presidents—have been writing about epidemics and pandemics for centuries, reflecting on what causes them, what might stop them, and how people have reacted to them. We have, collectively, accumulated an untold amount of source material of value not only to historians. We have accumulated a record of successes and failures that should be an aid to those working on epidemics and pandemics now.

Chapter 1
Plague

Plague. A word more freighted with meaning in the history of disease would be hard to find. It is a disease we now know to be caused by a bacillus, *Yersinia pestis*, transmitted by the bite of an infected flea—a flea seeking a human host after its animal host died. It first appeared in the sixth century CE when the first identifiable pandemic occurred during the Byzantine Empire. It is commonly called the Plague of Justinian after the eastern Roman emperor Justinian. Where it originated is uncertain—it possibly came from the interior of central Africa to Ethiopia and went on to Byzantium via well-established trade networks. But it might have come from Asia. We don't know. It first appeared in the historical record in 541 in the Egyptian port city of Pelusium. It took two years to travel the length and breadth of the Mediterranean, sparing no country along its coast, moving on to Persia in the east and the British Isles in the north.

Although precise demographic data does not exist, it is clear that the pandemic had devastating effects on mortality. John of Ephesus, in his *Ecclesiastical History*, detailed his encounter with the plague as he coincidentally traveled along its path from Constantinople to Alexandria and back through Palestine, Syria, and Asia Minor. He documented fallow fields, vineyards with grapes unpicked, animals gone feral, and people who spent their days digging graves. The Greek historian Procopius said that plague claimed ten thousand lives in Constantinople in a single day in 542. The "whole human race came near to being annihilated." Evagrius, another contemporary observer, thought the plague took three hundred thousand lives in the Byzantine capital. These numbers are impressionistic—an impression of deadly devastation. Procopius and other Greek observers of the plague familiar with earlier epidemics agreed that there had never been one like the Plague of Justinian. Pre-Islamic Arabic writers noted the novelty and reported that the plague had a major demographic effect on the eastern reaches of the Roman Empire. Early Islamic writers chronicled death on such a scale and at such a pace that it forced the abandonment of burial practices. When it finally reached mainland England in the mid-seventh century, Bede, in his *Ecclesiastical History*, lamented that plague's "sudden pestilence rag[ed] far and wide with fierce destruction...and carried off many throughout the length and breadth of Britain."

For more than two hundred years, beginning with the Plague of Justinian, more than a dozen separate epidemics visited parts of Europe and the Near East. By the end of the eighth century it was gone, perhaps no longer able to find susceptible human or rat hosts.

The plague's effects varied from place to place. On a grand scale, the effects of rural depopulation on the finances of the Byzantine Empire—effects gleaned from careful attention to numismatic, papyrological, and legal evidence—suggest that the first plague pandemic might have contributed to the downfall of the empire itself. By contrast, plague did not reach Britain until 664; it disappeared twenty-three years later. Its immediate impact—mass death, the emptying out of monasteries, the abandonment of villages—was shocking. Its long-term effects might well have been negligible. Northumbrian monastic life was hard hit by the plague in the 660s; two generations later it was thriving. Plague seems to have been no match for good land, royal power, and vast wealth. These conclusions are based on slivers of evidence, for when one tries to look beyond monasteries and into life more generally, documentation disappears.

The impact of the plague was keenly felt in the short and long term in Syria. Ships infested with plague arrived from Egypt in 542 at the ports of Gaza, Ashkelon, and Antioch. From there it traveled to Damascus, then spread south. We know from John of Ephesus that it was devastating. From then on, plague struck Syria every seven or so years between 541 and 749. In the short term, high mortality and mass flight left many places empty. Over the long term, repeated outbreaks had a deleterious effect on agricultural production and the populations of settled communities. The mobile lifestyle of Arabia prevented the plague from taking hold and in turn increased the power of nomadic populations. The continued fragility of agricultural production meant a reduction in crop-based taxes and the rise of a pastoral economy. So frequent was plague in Syria and so devastating were its effects by early Islamic times that Syria developed a reputation as a land riddled with plague. The impression stuck. By the medieval period Islamic Syria was well known as having had a long and disastrous experience with plague.

What we do not know about the first pandemic overshadows what we do. This may change as more sophisticated tools of analysis become available. Careful reading of textual sources can get us only so far. Historians will need to draw from disciplines such as zoology, archaeology, and molecular biology if the mysteries of the first pandemic are ever to be revealed.

Europe's apparently plague-free centuries came to an end in 1347 when plague returned and took with it up to half of the continent's population—perhaps more. When the first wave of the so-called second pandemic finally fled in 1353, it left in its wake a continent forever changed. After it reappeared in 1347 the plague regularly revisited much of Europe and the Islamic world. Its last European outbreak was in Russia in 1770. The second plague pandemic was not one event; it was a series of epidemics that varied in severity, scale, and scope. For decades, most scholars have believed that plague was introduced once from central Asia in the middle of the fourteenth century and then established a reservoir. Recent research into the correlation between changes in the climate in central Asia and epidemics of plague in Europe suggest that the old model might need revision. It is possible that plague came to Europe again and again. When the climate warmed, the central Asian gerbil population exploded and became a highly mobile, widespread host for fleas. The fleas would then jump to humans and domesticated animals, which would then transport them to Europe at a time of robust trade relations between Asia and European ports such as Dubrovnik.

Over the centuries Europeans adapted to the plague, even came to expect it, and developed ways of dealing with it. As a result, reactions to and consequences of plague in Florence in 1348 were different than they were for the 1665–66 plague in London, for example. Florence experienced a new and novel event; London, as cataclysmic as the plague might have been in the 1660s, experienced a familiar and increasingly well-understood disease. None of this was so during the first pandemic. No one was prepared; no one knew what was happening. It was novel and uniquely deadly. It was the Black Death.

For seven years plague swept across Europe, devastating the city and the countryside. It first appeared in the historical record in 1346 in the Black Sea port of Kaffa and spread inexorably across Europe. It demanded an explanation. How and why were so many people dying? The how was explained in several overlapping ways: providence, miasma, contagion, and individual susceptibility. As with cholera, these explanations—especially miasma and contagion—would dominate theories of disease transmission until nearly the end of the nineteenth century. During the Black Death—a time when the late medieval rediscovery of the writings of Galen and Hippocrates, via newly translated Arabic renderings of Greek and Latin texts, was in full flower, and the notion of bad air causing disease flourished—miasma and contagion were not as opposed to one another as they would become. People might become infected because of the miasmatic air seeping up out of the ground as rotting vegetable matter released its toxic gases. They would then be contagious and able to pass the disease on to others—especially those uniquely susceptible such as sinners and malcontents, the licentious and the gluttonous.

These earthly explanations for plague's path were subsumed in what most thought was the ultimate cause of the plague: God's wrath. Before plague reached him, Ralph of Shrewsbury, the bishop of Bath and Wells, implored his flock to pray. Toward the end of the summer of 1348 he wrote, "Since a catastrophic pestilence from the East has arrived in a neighboring kingdom, it is very much to be feared that unless we pray devoutly and incessantly, a similar pestilence will stretch its poisonous branches into this realm, and strike down and consume the inhabitants." Divine explanations were augmented by others. In one of the most detailed contemporary explanations, the masters of the faculty of medicine at Paris wrote in October 1348 that the "distant and first cause of this pestilence was and is the configuration of the heavens.... This conjunction, along with other earlier conjunctions and eclipses, by causing a deadly corruption of the air around us, signifies mortality and famines." When Jupiter and Mars, in particular, came together, this caused a "great pestilence in the air." Jupiter drew vapors out of the earth; Mars ignited them. But even with this scientific explanation, one driven by observation and theory and devoted to the notion that medicine played a role in controlling the disease, plague was still ultimately caused by God. "We must not overlook the fact that any pestilence proceeds from the divine will, and our advice can therefore only be to return humbly to God."

Many reacted in horror to the plague, as Giovanni Boccaccio so vividly documents in *The Decameron*. Based on Boccaccio's experience in Florence, *The Decameron* is an unparalleled literary representation of the plague's reception. Boccaccio was agnostic on the cause—it might have been the "influence of heavenly bodies," or it might have been "punishment signifying God's righteous anger at our iniquitous way of life." Whatever the cause, "in the face of its onrush, all the wisdom and ingenuity of man were unavailing....All of the advice of physicians and all the power of medicine were profitless and unavailing."

The misery caused by plague led people to abandon the laws of God and man; there were few left alive to enforce them. Those outside the city without medical care or family or community to take care of them, Boccaccio wrote, died "more like animals than human beings." Never before had such a calamity struck. "The cruelty of heaven (and possibly, in some measure, also that of man) was so immense and so devastating that between March and July of the year in question...it is reliably thought that over a hundred thousand human lives were extinguished within the walls of the city of Florence." A French observer noted that half the population of Avignon perished; in Marseilles four out of five were dead. As the disease traveled through France, the "scale of the mortality [meant] that for fear of death men [did] not dare speak with anyone whose kinsmen or kinswoman has died, because it has often been observed that when one member of a family dies, almost all of the rest follow." Suspicion and fear were rampant: family members treated their sick like dogs; neighbors shunned one another. In city after city the dead were buried en masse in plague pits that were an affront to established burial rituals and, at least in the short term, suggest a breakdown of order. Helpless in the face of such death, many chose flight, but in the Muslim world running from God's will was considered blasphemous. Some searched for scapegoats. Mobs wiped out perhaps as many as one thousand Jewish communities across Europe.

Despite the helplessness many felt, cities such as Venice and Florence responded by creating sanitary commissions. To ensure that the air was pure, they enforced the cleaning of sewers and the collection of garbage. When it seemed clear plague was on its way to Florence, the city forbade those traveling from Genoa or Pisa from entering. When plague did arrive, sanitary regulations sought to effect the removal of all "putrid matter and infected persons, from which might arise or be induced a corruption of the air." These measures were largely ineffective. Plague came and it killed. It would be a century or more before anything remotely effective could be put in place—and by then the virulence of the plague had diminished anyway.

People who lived through the Black Death reacted in numerous ways: they tried to explain the catastrophe; they reeled in horror; they ran away; they blamed outsiders. What is more difficult to discern are the longer term effects of the Black Death on demography, the economy, social customs, culture, religion, and so forth. In the near term, the plague decimated a significant portion of the population—one recent estimate is that 60 percent of Europe perished. Population stayed low for a century, leading to labor shortages, higher wages combined with inflation, and the opening of more land. Depopulation changed, for a time, some aspects of the social and economic order. This is best documented in England. In 1349, at Eynsham Abbey, the dearth of laborers forced the abbot and the lord of the manor to enter into a new labor agreement with the tenants with far more favorable terms. In 1351, the unfree peasants on the estate of John de Vere, Earl of Oxford, were relieved of many of their obligations. On yet another estate, the royal manor of Drakelow in Cheshire, rents were lowered by a third "due," according to the accounting official, John de Wodhull, "to the effects of the pestilence. The tenants threatened to leave (which would have left the lord's tenements empty) unless they were granted such a remission, to last until the world improves and the tenements came to be worth more." Wages went up, but so too did the cost of almost all basic goods—a demand for labor based on scarcity also meant a scarcity of goods. In response to demands for lower rents and higher wages,

Parliament passed the Ordinance of Labourers in 1349 and the Statute of Labourers in 1351 to set wage limits, compel people to work, and punish those who disobeyed. Facing a severe labor shortage, the government acted swiftly against those who attempted to take advantage of the crisis.

That laws against seeking higher wages and lower rents were necessary suggests that in the immediate aftermath of the Black Death and in the subsequent decades of the fourteenth century there was a perceptible change in *mentalité*. Elite commentary on the (much maligned) behavior of the peasantry bears this out. They used their newfound surplus to purchase clothes not befitting their station in life; they also increasingly took up hunting—once the exclusive enclave of the rich.

The poet John Gower lamented the passing of the old ways: "The labourers of olden times were not accustomed to eat wheat bread; their bread was made of beans and of other corn, and their drink was water. Then cheese and milk were a feast to them; rarely had they any other feast than this. Their clothing was plain grey. Then was the world of such folk well-ordered in its estate." But now "our happy times of old have been rudely wiped out." Because "servants are now masters and masters are servants... the peasant pretends to imitate the ways of the freemen, and gives himself the appearance of him in his clothes." Sumptuary laws directed at the "outrageous and excessive apparel of divers people against their estate and degree" also suggest that peasant behavior was markedly changing. Lamentations for times past, when people knew their station in life, were common in the decades after the Black Death. Despite the presence of laws forbidding both demanding and paying excess wages, the practice was common: in the face of a continued labor shortage, made worse by subsequent epidemics in 1360–62 and 1369, there was often no other choice.

Laborers in Italy demanded higher wages, too. In Florence, the chronicler Matteo Villani noted that "serving girls and unskilled women with no experience in service and stable boys want at least 12 florins per year, and the most arrogant among them 18 or 24 florins per year, and so also nurses and minor artisans working with their hands three times or nearly the usual pay, and laborers on the land all want oxen and all seed, and want to work the best lands, and to abandon all others." That these demands were more than the disgruntled wishes of a few is clear when one sees the official responses: attempts to cap wages and force people to accept employment no matter the terms.

Though it is difficult to get a grasp on precisely how standards of living might have changed—the data is hard, if not impossible, to come by—it does seem likely that both men and women in the decades after the Black Death, ironically, were better off than their counterparts in the decades of want preceding the plague.

Europe's demographic decimation was a short-term shock. Within a century much of the continent's productivity and population rebounded and even flourished. But it would take nearly two hundred years for pre-plague population levels to be reestablished over much of the western Mediterranean; it would not happen in England until after 1600. Yet the population decline did not have a long-term adverse effect. One possible explanation is that the pre-pandemic population might have reached a Malthusian critical mass where resources had reached their carrying capacity. In this view, the Black Death, while a tragedy in the short term, was perhaps, viewed over a longer time horizon, beneficial. The well-documented increase in real wages across all of Europe in the century after the Black Death might best be explained by the increased premium on labor. Attributing changes in the economy and demography of such a large swath of space to a single cause, no matter how devastating, is not possible. Even generalizations are hard to make. Many changes may have already begun taking place: population was declining here and there; in many places, labor relations and land tenure were undergoing change before the Black Death—serfdom disappeared from Flanders and

Holland in the twelfth and thirteenth centuries with no assistance from the plague at all. But on the other hand, it is possible that the Black Death jumpstarted a century and more of technological innovation. Power-generating devices such as wind and water mills proliferated; firearms did too. Were these tools a response to the dearth of bodies in the wake of the plague? Possibly. What seems undeniable is that if the plague was not the singular cause of change, it certainly was an accelerant.

A catastrophe of such a scale left a mark on literature, art, and worship. In the wake of the plague we see an excess of piety in some places, as well as rebellion against the strictures of the church. Central European flagellants—religious devotees who publicly performed their unique form of piety by whipping themselves, among other things—began taking on the conventional roles of the clergy and professing that Christ was on his way to earth to put an end to oppression by taking from the rich and giving to the poor. A fascination with the macabre in artwork suggests a newfound awareness of the unpredictability of mortality. Universities expanded in the plague's aftermath—a dearth of priests and the consequent lapses in learning brought on by the plague inspired their founding. In England, grand cathedral construction gave way to building smaller, more modest churches.

In the decades and centuries after the Black Death, doctors gained more confidence, mortality declined, and governments began to take a more active role in managing the plague. People became accustomed to plague as it became a regular feature of life in many places. London suffered seventeen outbreaks between 1500 and 1665. For nearly three hundred years—1500 to 1720—not a year passed in France without plague. In Egypt, it appeared every eight to nine years, and in Syria-Palestine there appear to have been eighteen major epidemics between the Black Death and the Ottoman takeover in 1517. Its regularity and the fact that there was never again a brutal and shocking continent-wide conflagration as devastating as the Black Death meant that there was much less fear and very little scapegoating; in contrast to the innumerable attacks on Jews during the Black Death, during the next century there was only one, in Poland. The extreme shock of the Black Death did not return; plague became horrifyingly normal. Medical doctors and municipalities gained confidence in their ability to confront it. While no one knew just when or where plague would come—it possessed, as one historian has put it, an "inexplicable randomness"—a broad pattern did begin to reveal itself: first, it struck ports; it next moved inland, and then from the city to the country. In cities, it appeared in some neighborhoods and not others; it moved from house to house, seemingly at random. Patterns of behavior became discernible. Flight was common. So was an urge for self-preservation that meant, at times, a disregard for others. Generally speaking, governments remained intact, and plague did not spell the end of the social order. Official responses to plague—government-sponsored health boards, hospitals, and pest houses, as well as the machinery of quarantine—strengthened the state across much of early modern Europe.

Methods of control changed as doctors less and less understood the origins of the plague to be found in God's wrath or the alignment of the planets. They sought more earthly explanations and they tried to cure it. By the end of the fourteenth century, and increasingly in the fifteenth, doctors began to see the plague as beneficial to their practice. The wealth of clinical experience that came from experimenting with various cures is well documented in a new genre of writing that emerged in the late medieval period devoted to explain plague: the plague tractatus. Because some epidemics were comparatively minor, people had time to get to know the disease in less anxious and terrifying circumstances than would have been possible during a major epidemic. The newfound confidence led many to claim that they had surpassed ancient masters such as Hippocrates and Galen, asserting that these former authorities had no experience with the disease they themselves now mastered.

After the Black Death, loss of life on such a scale was not seen again. There were serious epidemics—up to 60 percent of the population of Genoa perished in 1656–57, and at least six other outbreaks took upwards of 30 percent of the populations of places such as Marseilles, Padua, and Milan. Mostly, mortality declined. The marked reduction in mortality very clearly corresponds with the newfound confidence in medicine. Some of this confidence surely came with new understandings of the disease such as the need for isolation of patients. But it is also possible that the disease itself was becoming less and less severe as populations built up some immunity.

The idea of contagion has a long history. It followed a twisted path from Galen, who developed a theory of contagious seeds, to the Renaissance; along the way it stopped in the Arabic world, where it gained little traction over miasma and God; it began to catch on in Europe in the sixteenth century. The notion that plague might be contagious appeared as early as the late fourteenth century. Just as the Black Death was wreaking havoc in the Mediterranean, the Arabic writer Ibn al-Khatib offered one of the clearest declarations in favor of contagion. His views were in stark contrast with the more common Muslim belief that God sent plague. Ibn al-Khatib wrote, "If it were asked, how do we submit to the theory of contagion, when already the divine law has refuted the notion of contagion, we will answer: The existence of contagion has been proved by experience, deduction, the senses, observations, and by unanimous reports, and these aforementioned categories are the demonstrations of proof."

The theory of contagion that began to emerge in early modern Europe was often accompanied by miasma. And God was still very much present. Some, like the English preacher Richard Leake, had no tolerance for earthly explanations. He intoned, "It was not infection of the air, distemperature in men's bodies, much less the malicious and devilish practice of witches, or yet blind fortune, or any other such imagined causes, which were the breeders of these evils, but the mass and multitude of our sins." Plague was God's punishment. In the tiny village of Monte Lupo, in the Tuscan hinterlands, plague arrived in the fall of 1630. Secular and religious officials battled over its causes and cures. Religious leaders, along with most of the townspeople, wanted to placate God with a religious procession. Secular health officials, believing that plague was contagious, attempted to restrict such public gatherings and isolate the sick and their families. Riotous violence ensued. In Spain and Italy such authors as Francisco Valles, Vetorre Trincavella, and Girolamo Fracastoro suggested that diseases like plague passed from person to person. As Valles put it in his commentary on Galen's *Epidemics*, "No contagion or disease can occur without the transmission of something from the already infected person to the person who is being infected. That is agreed, since every natural action occurs by contact.... There are thus sent out seeds of contagion, which are some sort of defilements, from the sufferer to the person about to be affected by the contagion." But early modern views of contagion were very different than modern ones. Stephen Bradwell, an English commentator, writing in 1636, mixes contagion and miasma without compunction, for they are not, at this stage of explaining plague (and other diseases), mutually exclusive: as he wrote, "That which infecteth another with his own quality by touching it, whether the medium of the touch be corporeal or spiritual or an airy breath." The infectious agent was a "seminary tincture full of a venomous quality, that being very thin and spiritous mixeth itself with the air, and pierces the pores of the body."

The (incomplete) shift toward belief in contagion manifested itself in a move toward quarantine and isolation of both people and goods, travel restrictions, prohibitions on public gatherings such as religious processions, and a general increase of state power over the individual lives of the sick and suspected sick. In northern Italy, where these measures were pioneered, boards of health enforced laws regarding public health in times of plague. They had little effect; plague still came.

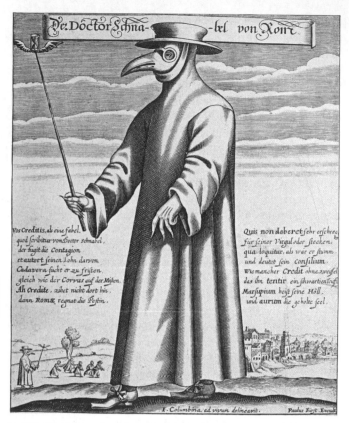

1. This 1656 engraving shows the iconic plague doctor wearing a protective mask filled with herbs to ward off the pestilence.

What they might have reflected and reinforced, however, was an emerging association between poverty and disease. It did not go unnoticed in Italy, France, and England that plague preyed more upon the poor than the rich. Writing during the last major outbreak of plague in Marseilles in 1720, one doctor had this to say about a wealthy neighborhood: "The streets are wide, the houses are large, and inhabited chiefly by persons in a state of opulence and such are always the last attacked by a contagion, on account of the means they have to place themselves out of its reach." At a time when many thought plague was contagious and a disease of the poor, the wealthy began to worry increasingly about its passage between the classes. Plague became a social problem. It took on meaning as a symbol of the divide between rich and poor. Fear of the plague and fear of the poor went hand in hand.

Plague's contagious nature also had an effect on commerce as European states sought to impose quarantine on goods. Maritime quarantine dates back to the late fourteenth century, when it was first imposed in the port of Dubrovnik. Over time it became routine, if controversial and not necessarily effective. Quarantine was not relegated to goods alone; people, too, could be, and often were, detained. The association between trade, travel, and the plague was longstanding. Because most believed that plague had come from the east and that it was in some way infectious, detaining goods and people from that part of the world had an appeal that was hard to resist. The same was not so in the Muslim world, where contagion was far less well accepted, and the administrative capacity necessary for quarantine did not exist in the Ottoman Empire. India and China, other commonly invoked sources of plague, did not practice quarantine either. It was thus up to European states, particularly in the Mediterranean, to police their own borders. The sense that disease arrived from the east and the belief that nothing was being done to curtail its movement would only hasten the divide between east and west—a divide that would grow stronger during the cholera pandemics of the nineteenth century.

Not all states adopted quarantine with equal vigor. Those that did were in closer proximity to the sources of plague. Just as important was the growing association between a state's ability to govern and its ability to keep its people free from epidemics. This association was most powerfully felt in the independent Italian city-states and was in full flower by the late sixteenth century when all of Italy was engulfed by the plague in 1575–78. Italy's efforts to control plague through improved sanitation, strict control over the movement of people and goods—especially from outside—increased knowledge regarding the source of an epidemic, and the creation of more and more sanitary boards where there had been none initially made Italy unique. But its methods began to catch on elsewhere in Europe—Italy's influence is evident in England's first plague orders from 1578—and quarantine and isolation, especially, became more and more common.

Despite these early efforts at state control over epidemics, the effects were often tempered by lax enforcement, porous borders, and the power of merchants to subvert restrictions on their livelihood. Further, the Italian city-states were small, with populations that for centuries had been devoted to civic pride and protection. Erecting such an edifice in France, which was much larger and more heterogeneous, proved challenging. Even when maritime quarantine was in effect, as it was in 1664 in London as plague made its way from the Low Countries, it did not always work, for that year and into the next two London suffered its worst epidemic in more than a century. In theory, household quarantine of the sick was a good idea; in practice it did little: plague victims disregarded orders to stay put, and there were simply too many of them. Quarantine as a public health measure and its effect on commerce would come under considerable fire in the eighteenth century as it increasingly began to seem like a holdover from a less enlightened time.

If the beginning of the second plague pandemic can be dated rather precisely to 1347 and the arrival of the Black Death, the same cannot be said about the final years of the pandemic. It petered out slowly, leaving one place and then another, never to return. Plague visited England for the last time in 1665–66, when it killed eighty thousand Londoners. Half a century later it made its last appearance in western Europe in Marseilles. Fifty years after that Moscow hosted the last European epidemic. It visited

Egypt over and over again throughout the eighteenth century, killing as many as 20 percent of Cairo's population of three hundred thousand during the major epidemic of 1791. It persisted in the Ottoman Empire well into the nineteenth century. For more than three centuries plague had affected religious beliefs and theories of disease transmission, as well as demography and the economy; it ushered in the first state-sponsored public health measures. And then it was gone. When looked at across the early modern world, plague appears to have gradually petered out—after all, it was more than a century between London's last epidemic and Moscow's. But when looked at locally or at the country level, it appears to have disappeared suddenly. England had been visited by the plague regularly since the 1340s. Then it made one last dramatic appearance in 1665–66 and never returned. The same is true of France: after centuries in which no year was plague-free, the epidemic in Marseilles in 1720 was the last. What happened? Rats may have developed immunity, stopping plague in its tracks, or perhaps the dominant species of rat changed. Perhaps the climate fluctuations in central Asia that might have reintroduced plague time and again ceased. Further, despite the fact that in many cases quarantine was not effective, it might be that over the long term it worked to gradually slow down the movement of the plague. After 1666 England began to strictly enforce quarantine; plague never returned. But because plague lasted for so long in so many diverse places and ended at different times, it is not possible to determine a single cause of the disease's demise.

When pandemic plague reappeared in the 1890s, historical memory had not vanished. The nineteenth-century experience with pandemic cholera reminded those countries that experienced plague what it meant to deal with epidemic disease; most of the strategies deployed against cholera had been developed during the second plague pandemic. Its influence loomed large. And so, in turn, did experience with pandemic cholera influence the ways in which the third plague pandemic would be managed.

The third pandemic began in southern mainland China in 1890. That year, plague spread along the Canton River, reaching Guangdong and then southern China's largest trading city, Guangzhou. From there it traveled the short distance to Hong Kong and beyond. For the rest of the decade the third pandemic spread around much of the world, concentrated mostly in port cities. Cape Town, Sydney, Honolulu, and San Francisco all experienced plague. So did Rio de Janeiro and Buenos Aires. In Oporto, Portugal, maritime quarantine stopped the city's commercial activity. And while mortality in these cities was relatively low, fear and panic were high—eighty thousand fled Hong Kong; in Cape Town and Sydney quarantine became a means to put into effect racial policies designed to manage the black African and Chinese populations; harsh measures were directed at the Chinese in San Francisco and Honolulu. Plague made its way across much of northern and western India, where it killed nearly twelve million people. Senegal fell victim to the third pandemic in 1914, and for the next thirty years plague challenged French colonial management of the country. In Manchuria in northeast China a deadly form of pneumonic plague broke out in 1910.

The third plague pandemic was not the return of the Black Death. With the important exception of India, mortality was much lower—the disease might have been less virulent, and public health measures were more robust. Surveillance systems, maritime quarantines, isolation of victims—all of these and more were put in place, sometimes with brutality and heavy-handedness, to contain plague. In Alexandria, Egypt, rather than forcing people to adhere to strict public health measures, health officials enlisted local leaders to gain the trust and cooperation of the citizenry. As a result, mass panic was avoided, and Alexandria's epidemic burned out in a few months.

The pandemic's fast course around much of the globe was made possible by rapidly developing global trade networks and human

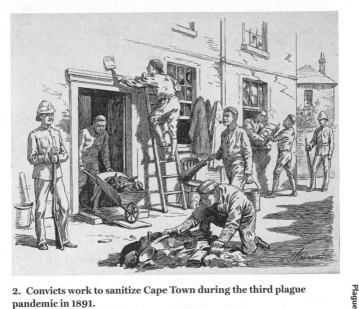

2. Convicts work to sanitize Cape Town during the third plague pandemic in 1891.

migration via ever faster steamships and an enormous increase in rail lines. The relationship between commerce, migration, and epidemic infectious disease—and the need to develop means of international cooperation to deal with the problem—had been evident throughout the nineteenth century as a result of pandemic cholera. The relationship became clearer when plague returned, and would be made so again in 1918 when pandemic influenza circled the globe.

Plague returned in the midst of the laboratory revolution. At the very beginning of the pandemic in 1894, Alexander Yersin, a Swiss-French scientist, and Shibasaburo Kitasato, a Japanese researcher, working independently, discovered the plague bacillus within ten days of each other. Next, as the pandemic made its way around the world, so too did the idea—first proposed by French scientist Paul-Louis Simond while working in Bombay in

1898—that plague was transmitted through fleas living on rats. Debates over who gets plague and why and how it was transmitted, which had preoccupied writing on the plague for centuries, came to an end.

Discovering the plague bacillus changed the identity of the disease. It did so in a very basic and rather sudden way: the plague that came back in the 1890s and was identified under the microscope in 1894 was a definite, knowable, if not quite tangible, thing; the disease that had been ravaging human populations since the sixth century had been unseeable and unknowable. After the identification of the bacillus this all changed, and the plague of the past turned into something identifiable in retrospect by its symptoms. Both Yersin and Kitasato claimed to have found the cause of the medieval plague. The modern, lab-based understanding of the disease would be imposed on the past. Before too long it was called *Yersinia pestis*.

The new way of seeing plague presented the problem of retrospective diagnosis. How can we know whether or not the disease that visited Constantinople in 542, Avignon in 1349, and London in 1665 was the same disease now known to be caused by *Yersinia pestis*? Some historians and biologists say they are not and stress possible differences in virulence; they claim that rats could not have traveled as fast as was necessary to spread the plague so quickly. They point to the absence of plague-like symptoms in some cases, and almost no evidence of mass rat death. Their case is built on differences between modern post-lab plague and premodern, pre-lab plague. The differences are stark enough that they cannot be the same disease.

Those who think that the two diseases are one and the same rely on similarities: the symptoms are the same, especially the presence of the telltale swelling in the armpits, groin, and the neck called buboes. It is almost certain that many, if not most, of the places that experienced plague in the past had considerable rat and flea populations. Like modern plague, plagues of the past—to the extent we can be certain—first made their way by sea, suggesting the agency of rats on ships. Also, supporters of the plague theory contend, the pathogen can change, and thus it is no surprise that plagues of the past looked different in some ways than the plague identified during the third pandemic. So what was the disease? By now, most historians, geneticists, and molecular biologists support the idea that the plague has always been *Y. pestis*. One reason for this is the emerging evidence from DNA sources originating in graves from antiquity, as well as from the late medieval and early modern periods.

Plague's relationship to commerce had of course been well known since its first appearance in the 1340s as a result of the Genoese trade with the east. From the 1850s to the end of the nineteenth century an emerging international community attempted to deal with the spread of infectious diseases at a series of regularly occurring International Sanitary Conferences. When the third plague pandemic arrived, scientific internationalism had reached an apex of sorts, exemplified by the International Sanitary Conference held in Venice in 1897, where the newest scientific knowledge about plague met a deep-seated desire for loose restrictions on trade. Science could serve commerce.

The Venice conference marked an unprecedented level of consensus on the part of the international community. The president of the London Epidemiological Society called the convention "a great advance on the part of the nationalities toward a truly *liberal* and truly *scientific* conception of the means to be adopted by respective governments for the prevention and control of infective diseases." Trying to contain the disease with quarantine fell by the wayside as more and more effective means of surveillance and reporting were put in place. If information about the plague's whereabouts was known, targeted responses such as immigration restrictions or port quarantines at the site of the outbreak could be launched rather than restrictive clampdowns inspired by fear and lack of knowledge. Not all nations adhered to the conference conventions—Portugal and Spain resorted to older, distinctly illiberal means such as ineffective military cordons around ports—but those that did, like Egypt, soon saw trade restrictions lifted. The consensus still held six years later, at a 1903 conference held in Paris. By then the focus had shifted to rats as the carrier of the disease, which in turn led to a focus on stopping plague at the ports of departure. This of course relied on both local capacity and interest in the two things most agreed were necessary to control plague: sanitary reform and a robust means of disease surveillance and notification. Across the world both of these policies were only unevenly in place.

The relationship between science and commerce was clear in India, far and away the country hardest hit during the third pandemic. From its arrival in Bombay in 1896, plague challenged the British colonial state's ability to manage the disease and called into question medical science's newfound confidence. The initial reaction was an unprecedented level of interference with and intervention into the daily lives of Indians, culminating in the 1897 Epidemic Diseases Act. The need to satisfy international demands that Britain stop plague from spreading to Europe gave colonial officials total power over shipboard inspections, neighborhood quarantines, restrictions on travel and religious gatherings, and sanitary measures. The act gave authorities license to try whatever they thought might work. This is turn gave medical science a newfound authority as colonial administrators allowed doctors and sanitary experts an unusual amount of influence over policy.

And those policies—fumigation and burning of houses; forcible removal to much feared hospitals where, among other things, caste conventions were not followed; forbidding funerary rituals; postmortem examinations; and the strict isolation of the sick— caused the greatest resistance to Western medicine in nineteenth-century Indian history.

The *Mahratta*, an English-language paper published in Pune, wrote that the British had never "interfered so largely and in such a systematic way with the domestic, social and religious habits of the people." One of the most hated practices, which spurred the most violent reactions, was family isolation, especially the removal of women to quarantine camps. In Pune, so resented was the practice of examining women in the streets and the frequent searching of houses by British soldiers that the plague commissioner, W. C. Rand, was assassinated in June 1897. The following year, after even more measures were put in place, resistance reached a head: rioting broke out all across northern India as a reaction to household searches, segregation, and hospitalization.

The colonial authorities were forced to relent—fighting the plague and the populace strained colonial capacities; the use of military force proved counterproductive. Perhaps working with rather than against the Indian population might be better. The sanitary commissioner came to realize that "experience is beginning to show that, what is medically desirable may be practically impossible, and politically dangerous."

After this change, even in Pune, where the most serious resistance had occurred, there emerged a spirit of cooperation between Indians and colonial officials. When the Indian Plague Commission issued a report in 1900, it noted that the shift from coercion to conciliation had been effective. What the resistance revealed and the new era of cooperation brought into stark relief was a lack of confidence in Western medicine, a realization that the British, despite their bluster, actually did not have the answers. Never again would they be able to impose their views on India in such a fashion. The suggestion that this was the dawn of an age of cooperation and equality would be belied by future developments in India. The point is that the British colonial authorities' initial handling of the plague revealed a state only capable of imposing its ideas by force. When that use of force backfired and the British were forced to come to terms with their failure, it was evident that the colonial state and Western medicine were not as powerful as they purported to be.

By World War I the third pandemic was either under control or burning out. But plague has not disappeared. Although it can now be treated with antibiotics, this must be done quickly, and because it is contagious it can spread fast. It has lingered for decades in parts of Africa and Asia; outbreaks in the 1990s in India and in the early twenty-first century in Madagascar remind the world that this ancient and feared disease still exists. But it has never again reached pandemic proportions.

Chapter 2
Smallpox

Until the World Health Organization declared the globe to be smallpox-free in 1980, it had been an endemic and pandemic disease for most of the last millennium, and possibly longer. Evidence from Egyptian mummies is tantalizing but not definitive; it is possible that the Plague of Athens, beginning in 430 BCE and so memorably described by Thucydides, was caused by smallpox. It has killed hundreds of millions of people. The earliest and clearest description of smallpox comes from the fourth-century Chinese alchemist Ho Kung, who wrote in what he called *Chou-hou pei-tsi fag* (Prescriptions for emergencies), "Recently there have been persons suffering from epidemic sores which attack the head, face and trunk. In a short time these sores spread all over the body. They have the appearance of hot boils containing some white matter. While some of these pustules are drying up a fresh crop appears." The most widespread description of the disease, which influenced clinical care into the seventeenth century, comes from the tenth century, when Rhazes, a Persian doctor based in Baghdad, wrote *A Treatise on the Small-Pox and Measles*. Evidence from China, India, and many parts of Africa demonstrates that smallpox has been a constant companion for centuries. Throughout much of northern India, especially in the eighteenth and nineteenth centuries, smallpox was considered a divine presence, not a disease. Sitala was the goddess of smallpox. The Cherokee, by the 1830s and perhaps sooner, had developed a dance called *itohvnv* designed to appease an evil spirit called Kosvkvskini thought to manifest in the form of smallpox. In West Africa, the Yoruba and others had a smallpox deity. In southern Africa, the Xhosa abandoned their funerary rites after a massive smallpox epidemic in the 1770s. No longer would they bury their dead; the infected died in the bush unattended. Death was no longer a natural, normal part of life but a feared and terrifying event. In Japan, the Ainu considered smallpox a god that transcended the boundary between the earthly and heavenly realms, turning people into ghosts who spread the disease among the living. It is no surprise that a disease that wreaked such havoc would have occupied a powerful place in the psyches of those it affected.

The African slave trade and settler colonialism brought smallpox to the New World, where it and other diseases reduced the indigenous population by as much as 90 percent. From the early sixteenth to the middle of the nineteenth century, as it continuously found a ready supply of susceptible hosts, smallpox caused a barrage of lethal epidemics across the hemisphere that morphed into a centuries-long pandemic.

Identifying the diseases present among the indigenous population of the Americas is challenging. Many sound similar, presenting with symptoms like fever, malaise, or a cough. Eyewitnesses could be maddeningly vague in their descriptions. However, because of smallpox's unique symptoms, most notably the pustules first described by Ho Chung, identifying it is less complicated than, for example, distinguishing between pneumonia and tuberculosis based solely on a colonial-era description. So clear were its symptoms to most contemporary observers—by the sixteenth and seventeenth centuries smallpox was a common childhood disease in much of Europe—that they called it by name rather than simply calling it a plague or a distemper. The Mexica had no word for a disease they had never seen before, but a description from 1520 in the Florentine Codex makes clear it was smallpox that had

Pandemics

decimated the Aztec capital Tenochtitlán and allowed for the Spanish takeover:

> There came amongst us a great sickness, a general plague. It raged amongst us, killing vast numbers of people. It covered many all over with sores: on the face, on the head, on the chest, everywhere. It was devastating. Nobody could move himself, nor turn his head, nor flex any part of his body. The sores were so terrible that the victims could not lie face down, nor on their backs, nor move from one side to the other. And when they tried to move even a little, they cried out in agony. Many died of the disease, and many others died merely of hunger. They starved to death because there was no one left alive to care for them. Many had their faces ravaged; they were pockmarked, they were pitted for life. Others lost their sight, they became blind. The worst phase of this pestilence lasted 60 days, 60 days of horror.

There is usually no mistaking smallpox for something else (though separating it from measles can be challenging).

How did a disease like smallpox, which was not especially virulent in Europe until the late seventeenth century, become such a killer in the Americas? Colonists in early New England thought God had brought death and disease to Indians as both a punishment for their heathen ways and a mechanism to clear the land. The Pilgrim chronicler William Bradford, reflecting on a 1633 smallpox epidemic, wrote, "It pleased God to visit these Indians with a great sickness." As a result, "God hath hereby cleared our title to this place." In Roanoke, Virginia, Thomas Hariot reported that the Algonquian thought that "it was the work of God through our means, and that we by him might kill and slay whom we would without weapons." The Huron blamed the French. According to a Jesuit missionary writing in the wake of a massive smallpox epidemic in the late 1630s, the Huron considered the French to be the "greatest sorcerers on earth," because everywhere the Jesuits went, Hurons died and missionaries lived.

Historians often ascribe catastrophic population loss to what are called virgin soil epidemics. The concept is simple: a disease that for many years had been a common childhood ailment in Europe became a population leveler amongst people with no previous exposure. Virgin soil can perpetuate the notion that somehow genetics and race combine to create populations that are weaker or stronger. That is not so. All populations are virgin soil until they are afflicted with a given disease. Smallpox ravaged the Khoisan of South Africa in a virgin soil epidemic in 1713; in Iceland, between 1707 and 1709, an epidemic killed nearly a third of this "virgin" population. All the concept tells us is that when a disease like smallpox arrived in a population that had a large number of non-immunes—initially, everyone in the New World; the Khoisan in the early eighteenth century; and much of Iceland at a time when there had been decades between epidemics—it could have catastrophic results. Virgin soil is an appealing explanation for American Indian susceptibility to diseases like smallpox. But it should be used only to explain the initial susceptibility to diseases not previously encountered.

Other factors help to explain smallpox's destructive path. There is the possibility that American Indian genetic homogeneity after millennia of isolation left them susceptible. It is possible, too, that much New World smallpox was of African, not European, origin and perhaps more virulent. Smallpox's continuous reintroduction into the New World, combined with a time lag between epidemics, meant that in many places when a new epidemic arrived, immune survivors from the previous epidemic were dead. Many populations were not large enough for smallpox to become endemic, providing them no chance to acquire immunity. (This same phenomenon helps to explain the devastating effects of smallpox among the pastoral populations of Kenya in the early decades of the twentieth century.) As long as a sufficient number of non-immunes remained in a community, smallpox thrived. Pregnant women who had never been sick could not pass on protective antibodies; mothers could not care for sick children when they themselves became sick. Many Indian communities were densely populated; further, large groups often shared a single dwelling—perfect conditions for the rapid spread of smallpox. Without any idea of contagion, the well visited the sick. Flight was common; smallpox spread.

The disruption caused by so much death left many to die of hunger and dehydration. In the 1630s, William Bradford wrote of the survivors of a smallpox epidemic that "the condition of this people was so lamentable and they fell down so generally of this disease as they were in the end not able to help one another, nor not to make a fire nor to fetch a little water to drink, nor any to bury the dead." Smallpox epidemics were a product of other calamitous developments of colonization. The Great Southeastern Smallpox Epidemic of 1696–1700 was made possible only by the disruption and constant movement brought on by the native slave trade—a trade that for decades disrupted native communities via raiding and migration.

Smallpox rearranged the ethnic landscape of native North America. For more than a century beginning in the 1630s, smallpox, spread by the European/native trade in beaver pelts, guns, and alcohol, wrought changes in the Great Lakes and the plains/prairie borderlands. Devastated by smallpox in the 1630s, the Iroquois increased their "mourning wars"—the capture of enemies to replace Iroquois dead—against their longtime foe, the Huron. Smallpox ravaged the Iroquois; it nearly decimated the Huron. And this, combined with Iroquois military prowess, allowed the Iroquois to emerge as the dominant power. The same epidemic forced the Sauk and Fox to seek refuge further west among other groups, fostering the creation of new ethnic identities. Smallpox kept coming and coming, rearranging the ethnic order again and again. Differential mortality left some groups weak and others strong. The Anishinaabe-speaking Monsoni, powerful middlemen in the beaver trade by the 1670s, were nearly wiped out by smallpox in the 1730s; survivors drifted to other groups, and by the end of the century they ceased to be a discrete people. Into the void stepped people like the northern Ojibwa.

In the early 1780s, a pandemic swept north out of Mexico City, reaching all the way to Hudson Bay and the Pacific Northwest. On the southern plains, once the shock subsided, the Comanche avoided smallpox: rather than travel to smallpox-ridden trade centers, they stayed put and waited for trade to come to them. Among other reasons, avoiding smallpox allowed them to become the most powerful, and largest, Indian people in the American West from the eighteenth to the mid-nineteenth century. On the northern plains, the pandemic nearly wiped out the villages along the Missouri River. The Arikara fell by as much as 80 percent. In 1795, the French trader Jean-Baptiste Truteau wrote: "In ancient times the Ricara nation was very large; it counted thirty-two populous villages, now depopulated and almost entirely destroyed by smallpox, which broke out among them at different times. A few families only, from each of the villages, escaped."

The balance of power tipped toward the equestrian peoples of plains—particularly the western Sioux, spared the worst of the pandemic through the blessing of geography. By 1800, the entire Great Plains region was dominated by horse-mounted hunters. The Missouri River villages had been decimated. As William Clark noted when he and Meriwether Lewis visited the plains in November 1804, "Maney years ago they lived in Several Villages on the Missourie low down, the Smallpox destroyed the greater part of the nation and reduced them to one large Village and Some Small ones, all [the] nations before this maladey was affrd. [afraid] of them after they were reduced the Sioux and other Indians waged war, and killed a great maney, and they moved up the Missourie."

Smallpox continued to torment Indians into the nineteenth century. The Mandan, Hidatsa, and Arikara on the Missouri River suffered an epidemic that nearly finished them off in 1837–38; the same epidemic moved west, leveling the Blackfeet, the Gros

Ventre, and the Assiniboine. Coming to fill the void was the increasingly powerful alliance of the Lakota, Cheyenne, and Arapaho. As the expanding American people moved further and further west in the mid-nineteenth century, the Indian world they found, a world dominated by the Comanche, the Lakota, the Arapaho, and the Cheyenne, was a world created by smallpox.

In early modern Europe smallpox was a familiar foe, endemic in many places, flowering into epidemics and pandemics in others. Before the middle of the seventeenth century, smallpox was not an especially virulent killer. It was a low-level endemic disease rarely written about as dangerous in medical texts or the accounts of chroniclers and travelers. There were no major epidemics. In places like late-sixteenth-century London, few died of the disease, and those few were children. Then, somehow, smallpox changed. By the eighteenth century it had become the continent's major killer, surpassing the plague in the public imagination and mortality. Beginning in 1649, and recurring at regular intervals for the rest of the century, smallpox epidemics became responsible for more than 8 percent of annual deaths in London. By the middle of the eighteenth century that figure had doubled: in 1762 smallpox claimed 3,500 people and was responsible for 17 percent of London's mortality. By the end of the century smallpox claimed between 8 and 20 percent of the population.

Inoculation, and later vaccination, began to change that. Inoculation involved introducing a small amount of the disease into a cut to induce a low-level reaction. If all went well, the patient would experience a mild form of smallpox and would become immune for life, just as anyone who had caught disease and survived. Inoculation had been practiced in parts of Africa, India, and China long before it became common in Europe in the middle of the eighteenth century. News of its effects trickled into England and the United States at the beginning of the century—in Boston, Reverend Cotton Mather reported that one of his slaves from West Africa had told him that it was common; news of inoculation from China arrived in England in 1700; and word that peasants from Poland and Denmark were inoculating in the seventeenth century began to spread. It caught on in the 1720s after Lady Mary Wortley Montague, the wife of the British ambassador to Turkey, had her daughter inoculated in 1718 in Constantinople, where the practice was well-known; in 1721 her son was the first person in Britain to be inoculated. Royal inoculations soon followed, and it became a common feature of British medical practice.

There was opposition, however: worry that infecting people with smallpox was dangerous, and concern in religious quarters that it interfered with fate. Most objections met with fierce rebuttal: inoculation saved lives by increasing the number of those immune to the disease. By mid-century it had become firmly established across much of western Europe and the Americas. Improvements in method, combined with the inoculation of entire villages and towns rather than just individuals, had an increasing effect on public health over the last half of the eighteenth century. Big cities like London were much harder to inoculate than small rural towns; they continued to suffer from smallpox. Inoculation changed the way people saw smallpox: it became a disease that had a specific, efficacious tool to fight it with. This smoothed the way for one of the most important breakthroughs in medical history: vaccination.

In 1796, when Edward Jenner prevented smallpox in a young English boy by inoculating him with a small amount of cowpox, rather than human smallpox via variolation, it signaled the beginning of the end. (The term "vaccine" comes from Jenner, who called cowpox *variolae vaccinae*, or smallpox of the cow.) Two years later he announced his discovery to the world. While others had inoculated with cowpox before him, Jenner's innovation was *proving* that it worked by subsequently infecting a patient with smallpox and demonstrating immunity. Vaccination with attenuated cowpox was quickly accepted as superior to inoculation with smallpox: there was no risk of catching smallpox, which meant no risk of spreading it. Within three years of Jenner's announcement a hundred thousand people in England had been vaccinated. Millions more followed over the next two decades: two million in Russia and nearly the same number in France. By 1800 vaccination had arrived in North America; the following year it arrived in Baghdad, and from there it went to India. By mid-century, smallpox's ravages dwindled among American Indians. Vaccination with cowpox (and variolation before it with smallpox) helped reduce the death toll. By the 1830s, the Hudson's Bay Company had vaccinated good portions of the native population of western Canada; in Guatemala colonial doctors began to inoculate the Maya in the 1770s, even adopting Mayan medical techniques like the use of obsidian knives. In the United States, vaccination efforts among American Indians were generally too little, too late—hence the horrible epidemic on the Missouri. Even so, as more and more people acquired immunity and the disease was introduced less and less frequently, the death toll declined.

In Japan, vaccination initially received a skeptical, even hostile, reception from a country that was previously "closed." Those who imported vaccine to the country were in the vanguard of opening Japan to the West; vaccine was a principle conduit for modernity. By the 1850s vaccine had been accepted. The Tokugawa Shogunate attempted to use a state-sponsored vaccination campaign to help make the Ainu less "primitive" and more Japanese. Whether that project was entirely successful is debatable. But what is clear is that long-held Ainu beliefs regarding curing smallpox could no longer be maintained in the face of vaccine. A whole belief system was rendered ineffective in the face of this new and effective procedure. In Europe, despite some early opposition from those who thought the practice dirty or doubted the existence of a single disease organism able to be stopped by another, vaccination spread, especially as it became compulsory in some places. In Sweden there were twelve thousand smallpox deaths in 1800. In 1822 there were eleven.

The European population climbed as mortality from smallpox declined.

Despite the early success of vaccination, major smallpox epidemics still erupted on several occasions, for once vaccination had reduced smallpox to such low levels, the initial zeal wore off, and so did its effects: though no one knew it initially, vaccination did not necessarily confer lifelong immunity. Between 1836 and 1839 thirty thousand died from smallpox in England. The pandemic of 1870–75—sparked by the Franco-Prussian War—killed an estimated five hundred thousand people and snapped much of Europe out of its slumber. England and Germany passed compulsory vaccination laws. In England, however, debate over the cause of diseases—environment, contagion, miasma—along with a powerful distaste for state intrusion into English bodies and a sense that smallpox had diminished in importance led to vociferous and at times violent opposition to compulsory vaccination. Various provisions of the Vaccination Acts of 1885 were overturned in 1898 and 1907.

Despite complacency regarding vaccination and the regular appearance of local outbreaks, the 1870–75 European pandemic was the last major appearance of smallpox on the continent. Vaccination, as well as the gradual replacement of variola major by variola minor—which is less contagious and less severe—meant that by the mid-twentieth century smallpox ceased to be a major problem in Europe, the United States, and much of the rest of the developed world. When the US Public Health Service recommended abandoning routine vaccination in 1971, it was because more children were dying—six to eight per year—from vaccine-related complications than were perishing from smallpox.

Vaccination against smallpox was a monumental public health achievement. It is an intervention that targeted an individual's health *and* had a profound effect on the public's health. Reducing the number of susceptible people in a population to a number insufficient to allow an infectious disease to spread is the key to controlling it. Earlier measures geared toward the public's health, like the use of quarantine during times of plague, were very different. Quarantine aimed to stop the spread of the disease during a particular epidemic; vaccination reduced the possibility that an epidemic would occur in the first place. Once enough people had been vaccinated, smallpox, with no non-human host, had no place to go.

Smallpox is the only human infectious disease humans have eradicated. The last case of variola major was in Bangladesh in 1975; two years later variola minor made its last appearance, in Somalia. A little more than a decade after embarking on an intensified eradication campaign in 1967—something the World Health Organization had initially been reluctant to do, instead deciding to try to eradicate malaria and failing—the WHO declared the planet smallpox-free in 1980. By almost any measure—the cost; the logistical, political, and social challenges; and the humanitarian effects—it was a colossal accomplishment.

Alone among infectious diseases, smallpox was an ideal candidate for eradication. A freeze-dried vaccine had been developed in the late 1940s, which meant that the challenge of deploying vaccine in tropical climates had been theoretically surmounted. The telltale rash made it easy to spot. Isolation and surveillance, methods pioneered in the early 1970s by the WHO's Smallpox Eradication Program (SEP), worked to stem its spread. No animal reservoir existed. Unlike malaria, carried by mosquitoes, there was no vector to consider when contemplating eradication, obviating the need for large-scale environmental manipulation. The push for eradication garnered widespread international support, allowing the WHO to intensify its efforts—before the newly ramped-up campaign began in 1967 smallpox eradication existed, more or less, in name only; it was a poorly funded and inadequately staffed afterthought at the WHO.

But why eradication? Smallpox had been declining since the introduction of Jenner's vaccine. While still present in some countries, it was not the most pressing health problem in many places. Intensifying the focus on smallpox lessened the focus on the conditions that gave rise to diseases in the first place. In places where it was still present but not a significant concern, like much of Latin America, eradication seemed to some an unnecessary distraction from more serious health matters, as well as being an enormous financial burden. The United States alone spent $1 billion in today's dollars on the SEP. But it was the countries where the campaign took place that were responsible for the majority of the costs. Still, where it caused the most mortality, in parts of Africa and South Asia, smallpox claimed two million people per year.

Once the WHO launched the intensified campaign, progress was rapid. Within a few years the number of countries with endemic smallpox shrunk to four—India, Bangladesh, Pakistan, and Ethiopia. Smallpox was most intransigent in India, and that is where the WHO launched its largest campaign. Even there the SEP made rapid, though not necessarily smooth or conflict-free, progress. Coercion and intimidation fostered by the campaign's alliance with Indira Gandhi's authoritarian regime; friction between Indian authorities and the WHO, as well as between local officials and the Indian government; problems with supplies and the quality of vaccine—all these things and more made the campaign in India especially challenging. Still, by 1975 India was smallpox-free.

The SEP was a success. But it should not be remembered as the work of top-down planning emanating from Geneva. The campaign involved countless local people whose input was seen by all as essential; frequent international meetings helped to

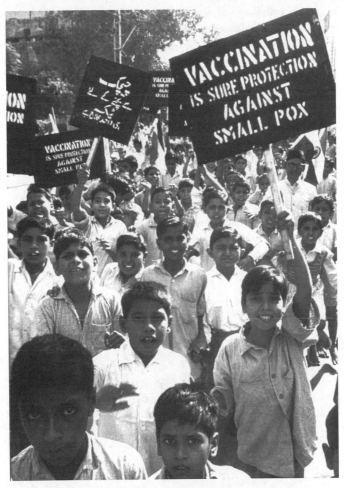

3. Indian children support the WHO and Indian government's
Smallpox Eradication Program in the 1950s. Public acceptance of the
effort was critical to its success.

encourage collaboration, share ideas, and learn from the myriad ways in which smallpox was and was not being controlled. To think of the smallpox campaign as successful solely because of the efforts of a few heroic individuals marshaling their troops or the work of the WHO would be a disservice to all those involved. It would provide a false lesson from the past, masking what the campaign really was: a multilevel, international, and indigenous effort that was responsive to often complex local conditions. Simplistic tales do no one any good.

Live smallpox now exists solely in secured labs, secreted away during the Cold War by the United States and the former Soviet Union. But in June 2014, two vials of viable smallpox DNA were found in an unused National Institutes of Health storage room, forgotten there for decades. This discovery briefly reminded the world of this once virulent, much feared killer.

Chapter 3
Malaria

Malaria originated in Africa and is caused by an infection with a parasitic protozoan of the genus *Plasmodium*. Throughout most of history, four types have infected humans: falciparum, malariae, ovale, and vivax. Recently, in Southeast Asia, as humans come into more and more frequent contact with primates due to deforestation, *P. knowlesi* has been causing malaria at an accelerating pace. The most common kinds are *P. falciparum* and *P. vivax*. *P. falciparum* is more lethal and dangerous. It is responsible for the vast majority of global malaria deaths.

Malaria might have existed in our hominid ancestors five million years ago. But because of the complicated lifecycle of the parasite, for an epidemic to occur a number of conditions must be met that provide the environment in which a sufficient number of mosquitoes and their human hosts can meet. Because it so often kills its host and does not live long in the human body—unlike tuberculosis, which can remain dormant for a lifetime after infection—malaria needs a constant resupply of hosts. This requires a dense population, which emerged slowly when the forests of central Africa began to be cleared for agriculture four to ten thousand years ago. Lots of mosquitoes are required. And mosquitoes need particular living conditions: those made available when farmers cut down vegetation and cleared the absorbent soil, creating pools of water ripe for mosquito breeding.

With few livestock available as hosts, mosquito species like *Anopheles gambiae* evolved to prefer humans for their blood meal. To spread, a malaria-experienced population must meet one that is immunologically naive.

Knowledge of malaria's early spread beyond Africa is scant. Solid evidence appears in much of the world after the first millennium BCE as malaria followed agriculture and human-induced environmental change. The region around Rome became malarious in the era of the late republic when economic conditions forced peasants to abandon low-lying farmlands, which then accumulated water and were transformed into marshy, malarial wetlands. Deforestation and the crumbling remains of a once vibrant drainage system added to the mix. From then until the middle of the twentieth century, southern Italy was malaria's European stronghold.

Malaria spread across early modern Europe alongside agricultural development. Its reach expanded during the era of the Atlantic slave trade from the late fifteenth century until the middle of the nineteenth century. It was during the seventeenth and eighteenth centuries, when the slave trade was at its height, that malaria from tropical Africa made its way into the New World tropics.

To thrive, malaria, like tuberculosis, needs human manipulation of the environment. Urban conditions gave rise to TB; those conditions that smoothed the way for malaria were largely rural and agricultural. The expansion of urban centers and agricultural production are related: the growth of cities fueled growth in agriculture. One can see this pattern in sixteenth- and seventeenth-century England, where a growing population and increased urbanization intensified agricultural production. In the Fenlands of southeastern England this led to draining some areas and creating marshes in others—conditions perfect for mosquitos and malaria. Malaria flourished as a steady influx of new peasant farmers provided susceptible human hosts.

Not all agricultural production is the same. Generally, where intensively capitalized agriculture took off—in the global north of the United States and parts of western Europe—agricultural improvement followed. In England, this meant ever more sophisticated methods for draining water, as well as out-migration of the rural population to cities, which reduced the number susceptible to malaria and capable of transmitting it. In the less developed global south, agricultural improvement was not as widespread; malarious conditions persisted; and a susceptible population remained.

Agricultural and rural development have been generally responsible for the proliferation of malaria, but poor urban sanitation and the presence of stagnant water can make malaria an urban disease—something that is happening more and more in the megacities of the global south. Other human-created environments also foster malaria. In the Panama Canal Zone in the early twentieth century, the mosquito most responsible for spreading malaria—*A. albimanus*—thrived in the conditions created by the canal's construction. An entomologist noted at the time: "*Anopheles albimanus* is closely associated with man and finds its most congenial surroundings about his habitations and in conditions he creates in the course of agricultural, engineering and other work." Joseph LePrince and A. J. Orenstein, authors of *Mosquito Control in Panama* (1916) noted that malaria "develops most rapidly when the soil is disturbed by large and extensive excavations and fills accompanied by the introduction of non-immune labor housed near the site of their work."

Following in the wake of agricultural settlement and the introduction of slavery, malaria wreaked havoc from the Chesapeake to the Mississippi valley to the Caribbean and beyond to South America. Exactly when malaria first arrived is unknown—perhaps early English settlers brought malaria (*P. vivax*) to the Chesapeake from southern England. By the middle of the seventeenth century African slaves had introduced

P. falciparum. It thrived among the non-immune settlers and their indentured servants across the New World tropics. When it seemed that enslaved Africans were less susceptible, they replaced indentured Europeans as a source of labor. The slave trade not only imported unfree labor into the Americas; it brought the epidemiological zone of tropical Africa to the New World.

Just as with cholera later in the nineteenth century and plague earlier, physicians in the tropics in the eighteenth century wondered if disease was a product of place or if it traveled. Many of these questions became tangled up with race and slavery. Noting different mortality rates, many wondered if Europeans were fated to die from tropical diseases while African slaves continued to resist them. It was a confounding question. As Dr. Robert Collins wrote of malaria and yellow fever in 1811 in his *Practical Rules for the Management of Negro Slaves in the Sugar Colonies,* "The reason why Negroes escape their fury, in the worst seasons, and most unhealthy situations, while whites die in great numbers, is a problem which no person has hitherto attempted to solve." Some argued that Europeans would adapt. In his classic text on the subject, *An Essay on the Diseases Incidental to Europeans in Hot Climates* (1786), James Lind wrote, "By length of time, the constitution of Europeans becomes seasoned to the East and West Indian climates.... Europeans, when thus habituated, are generally subject to as few diseases abroad, as those who reside at home." Did this mean there might be a universal human race, equally adaptable to the climates and diseases they lived among? Did climate determine biology? In the eighteenth century many thought the answer was yes.

Beginning in the nineteenth century, ideas about race began to change; the idea that climate determined health and that one would adapt began to disappear. Race became a fixed and hard boundary between peoples, and European optimism about settling the tropics was replaced by a set of rigid ideas about tropical places and "tropical races." In this way, malaria in the tropics contributed to the racialization of medicine.

After its initial appearance in the tropics in the seventeenth century, malaria was pushed ever inland via the varying forces of human migration. In the United States, an agricultural and malaria frontier moved west into the Ohio and Mississippi valleys. In Brazil, gold mining drew labor and malaria into the hinterlands. Massive forest clearing soon followed to make way for the vast farms needed to feed the new labor force—more than one million African slaves came to the interior during the so-called mining century of the 1700s. This new environment created the perfect habitat for one of *P. falciparum*'s most efficient vectors, *Anopheles darling*; the sedentary mining population provided the perfect hosts. Malaria exploded. But while malaria remained a problem into the twentieth century in the American South, the pattern established in places like England repeated itself: improvements in agriculture tended to reduce the burden of malaria, as these brought with them better housing and nutrition alongside decreased exposure. But in the tropics, malaria worsened and became a "natural" part of the region.

For much of the nineteenth century, malaria, along with cholera, was the quintessential miasmatic disease, brought on by the gases emitted from rotting remains of vegetable and animal waste; rain or other disturbances of the soil such as agricultural or urban development could contribute to the onset of these gaseous emissions. Its name even means bad air. Germ theory changed that. After Alphonse Laveran detected the malaria parasite in human blood in 1880 and continuing advances in the technology of pathology allowed more and more people to literally see, and thus accept, that malaria was caused by a protozoan, miasma theory no longer prevailed. Next came the vector. Near the end of the century, in 1898, Ronald Ross in India and Giovanni Grassi in Italy proved that anopheline mosquitoes transmitted malaria.

Malaria, like cholera and TB before it and plague shortly after, went from a disease explained by many things to a disease explained by one thing—the bite of an infected mosquito. The result: vector and parasite control, rather than mitigating the social or economic conditions that gave rise to malaria, prevailed.

Vector control worked—in places where mosquitoes were relentlessly attacked with sufficient resources or where the problem of malaria was limited. In the Panama Canal Zone at the turn of the twentieth century, William Gorgas, the colonel in charge of the United States' effort to render the Zone healthy, attacked malaria and yellow fever with unprecedented zeal by devoting himself to understanding the breeding habits and locales of mosquitoes and then destroying them. The abundant resources of the United States made this all possible. Within two years yellow fever disappeared. Malaria took longer—the reservoir of infection was greater, because it is possible to be reinfected with malaria (surviving yellow fever, by contrast, grants lifelong immunity). But malaria eventually succumbed.

Gorgas's success in Panama was a public health triumph lauded as an essential step toward the civilized settlement of the tropics. In "The Conquest of the Tropics for the White Race," published in 1909 in *Journal of the American Medical Association*, Gorgas considered the work he and others had done in Panama as the "earliest demonstration that the white man can flourish in the tropics and as the effective starting point of the effective settlement of these regions by the Caucasian." Optimism like this overturned the conviction that had prevailed throughout much of the nineteenth century that the tropics were unsuited to the white race.

The discoveries that led to the possibility of controlling malaria fostered a new field of medical inquiry—tropical medicine— devoted to understanding parasites and their vectors. Malaria led the way. According to tropical medicine's founder, Patrick

Manson, it was "by far the most important disease…in tropical pathology," because it was "the principal cause of morbidity and mortality in the tropics and sub-tropics." This new field spawned training programs, journals, and a research agenda. Schools of tropical medicine—the Liverpool School of Tropical Medicine was first, opening in 1897—were founded across Europe and the United States. A potent mix of optimism and hubris brought on by the very real breakthroughs in malaria control and the growing sense that diseases could be fought through modern medicine fueled the creation of tropical medicine. Malaria control was urgent, for in many places the disease was only getting worse as epidemics continued in the wake of uneven development.

Malaria declined where agricultural improvements reduced mosquito habitat and improved quality of life meant exposure to malaria was less frequent. But in many parts of the world peasant farmers had, and have, little opportunity to escape malaria and many chances to catch it. Peasant-based, undercapitalized farming left many people poor and continuously exposed. Large-scale plantation agriculture, focused on a single crop and employing the rural poor, often created the conditions for the spread of malaria: the destruction of forests for farms created perfect breeding grounds for mosquitoes. Since large plantations demanded lots of labor—labor not always available locally—a market in rural migratory labor emerged. Just as the forced labor migration of the Atlantic slave trade brought malaria to the New World tropics, labor migration in parts of Africa, South America, and Asia in the nineteenth and twentieth centuries introduced the disease into once malaria-free zones when workers recruited from areas with no malaria returned home and brought the disease with them. It was "the opening of the tropics" to large-scale, irrigation supported agriculture, according to C. A. Bentley and S. R. Christophers in their *The Causes of Blackwater Fever in the Duars* (1908), that turned malaria into an epidemic disease in India beginning in the 1860s. Where the soil drained poorly, irrigation canals became stagnant pools perfect for malaria breeding; the large tea estates attracted an enormous migrant labor force. It was the perfect scenario for spreading epidemic malaria.

Labor migration has been responsible for malaria epidemics at many times and in many places. For example, plagued by drought and left poor by sharecropping, the peasants of Brazil's semi-arid Sertão region—mostly malaria-free—migrated to the coast and to the Amazon for work. There they contracted malaria, brought it back home, and sparked outbreaks. An extended drought began in 1936, forcing greater and greater numbers of men to flee to find work. At the coast they confronted a virulent strain of malaria brought on by the recently introduced *A. gambiae*—accidentally imported by ship from West Africa. Those who survived the coastal epidemic returned to the Sertão, alongside migrants from the Amazon with still more malaria, and sparked a major malaria epidemic. The death toll was immense: officially five thousand, but likely more. A newspaper reported that the "human language is far from adequate to describe the desolation which existed in the region.... The general belief was that the Northeast would be depopulated because those who did not die at once would abandon it."

The arrival of *A. gambiae* combined with a susceptible population that was forced to migrate because of social and economic conditions caused the epidemic. In the 1920s and 1930s, likewise, forced migration of black South Africans from the malaria-free high veld into the malarious low veld created a new malarial population. And when they migrated back to the highlands to work on plantations set up by the very people who had displaced them, they brought malaria with them. With the spread of similar conditions showing no signs of stopping across much of the tropical world, a solution was necessary.

Those who wished to control malaria were split into two camps favoring different strategies: killing the mosquito vector or dealing with the infection from the plasmodium parasite. Gorgas's success in Panama and Cuba buoyed vector control, while controlling the parasite was made possible because of the discovery of the prophylactic quinine. Each had virtues and drawbacks. Quinine's limited value as a prophylactic was partly made up for by its therapeutic benefits. It worked to take care of symptoms, but supplies could be erratic and were expensive on a mass scale; its awful taste discouraged use. Plus, it did not stop transmission. That is, a person could be infected with the plasmodium, their symptoms stopped by quinine, but still able to spread the disease. Vector control worked. But it was expensive and logistically complicated. It demanded resources many places were unable to marshal. Neither addressed the underlying causes of malaria's continued presence.

After stunning success in several places, vector control prevailed. Gorgas might have been the pioneer, but there were other examples of successful vector control, such as the form known as species sanitation, which targeted specific *Anopheles* breeding grounds. Pioneered by Malcolm Watson in Malaya and then refined by N. R. Swellengrebel in Indonesia in the years just before World War I, this method of vector control was very effective. In Italy during the 1920s and 1930s, Mussolini's Fascist regime weakened malaria's grip by draining the Pontine Marshes, reclaiming them for agriculture, and resettling the area. In Palestine a smaller program of agricultural improvement and vector control brought malaria to its knees. And during the Great Depression in the United States, the Tennessee Valley Authority embarked on a program of rural betterment that involved ridding the region of malaria. Lowering water levels of dam-created reservoirs to desiccate *A. quadramaculatus*'s eggs, screening doors and windows (a practice more and more widespread since the nineteenth century), applying larvicides to breeding areas, and creating cattle grazing zones along shorelines to afford mosquitoes an alternative host all ensured the steady decline of malaria in the US South.

Vector control's place at the top of malaria mitigation efforts solidified in the years surrounding and including World War II. Breakthroughs in understanding the ecology of anopheline mosquitoes, especially increased knowledge about which species did and did not carry malaria; the success of Fred Soper and the Rockefeller Foundation at eradicating *A. gambiae* from Brazil; the discovery of the pesticide DDT during the war; and the same postwar impulse that spread TB control around the world all combined to make vector control triumphant. Malaria joined TB and smallpox as targets of the newly formed WHO's postwar global health agenda.

Malaria control was tied to the goal of fostering democracy and capitalism and stemming the tide of communism. The United States International Development Administration declared in 1956 that malaria control was easing urban overcrowding in Java and opening up Viet Minh–controlled areas to DDT spraying teams, and ridding the countryside of malaria in the Philippines meant that previously landless peasants could now become successful farmers on newly reclaimed land—and this is turn kept them from becoming Huk terrorists. Control of malaria meant the control of communism and the spread of democracy. The notion that "malaria blocks development"—that it meant the difference between becoming modern and economically well-developed or remaining poor and mired in tradition—was common. Malaria expert Paul Russell put it succinctly: malaria helped "to predispose a community to infection with political germs that can delay and destroy freedom." Biomedicine was for some, like American TB expert Walsh McDermott, the key to progressing in the modern world. "The biomedical goal of international development, or purposeful modernization, is to modify the disease pattern of an overly traditional society to a disease pattern that will not act as a major drag on a modernization effort."

So great was optimism surrounding the control of malaria that the WHO decided to eradicate it. Just as malaria became the archetypal tropical disease, it also became the disease that defined this era of hubris and overoptimism. Because of the abundant biomedical advances, especially antibiotics and DDT, it seemed like the time to think about ridding the world of some diseases. This was the climate in which infectious disease specialist T. Aidan Cockburn claimed in *Science* in 1961 that "we can look forward with confidence to a considerable degree of freedom from infectious diseases at a time not too distant in the future."

Malaria became a natural candidate for eradication. Knowing more and more about both mosquito breeding patterns and just which species transmitted malaria, having a demonstration of the power of eradication from Brazil, and being armed with an agent designed to kill the insect vector—all of these joined in the powerful postwar push into the developing world and added up to an unprecedented assault on malaria. Also important was that in 1955, when the WHO officially announced the Malaria Eradication Program (MEP), the global health bureaucracy was much smaller than it is today. The number of experts was comparatively tiny; many were like-minded; and most were members of the WHO's Expert Committee on Malaria. A very small group decided to eradicate malaria via indoor residual spraying with DDT. The major players were the WHO and donor governments like the United States; organizations such as UNICEF played important supporting roles. Funding largely came from the United States and such UN agencies as UNICEF; local governments covered the remaining amount—often at great sacrifice for what amounted in some cases to little gain.

The confidence with which the WHO embarked on the MEP was, it turned out, misplaced. Over the fourteen-year lifespan of the MEP, malaria proved far harder to eradicate in practice than theory suggested it should have been. After some early success in places like Venezuela, within a decade the program was faltering. Despite Africa having the vast majority of the world's malaria cases, the MEP, other than in a few demonstration projects, did

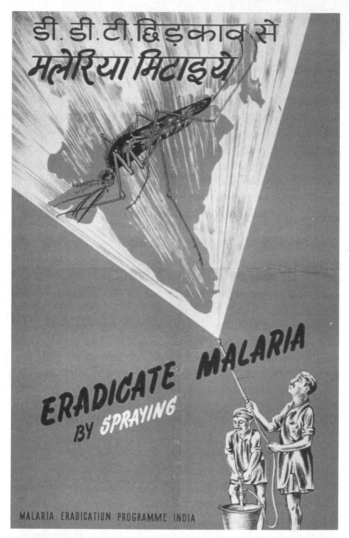

डी. डी. टी. छिड़काव से
मलेरिया मिटाइये

ERADICATE MALARIA
BY SPRAYING

MALARIA ERADICATION PROGRAMME INDIA

4. All over the world during the 1950s, the WHO's malaria eradication campaign was well publicized through commemorative stamps, posters (like the one here), radio campaigns, and other forms of propaganda.

not even attempt to rid it of malaria. The infrastructure was too weak and the problem too great; eradication on the continent would be impossible. So no one tried. In India the sheer size of the country, an unwieldy MEP staff of more than 150,000, the lack of basic healthcare throughout most of the country, and the growing problem of DDT resistance all added up to the conclusion that eradication was impossible.

In other places, like Brazil, the eradicationist impulse clashed with an already working program of malaria control. But the global health leadership at WHO, the Pan-American Health Organization, and the United States, as the major donor, remained wedded to eradication. In Brazil and Mexico, which were more or less forced to accept eradication, initial success with the program was met with later failures: when the MEP pulled out and mosquitoes (inevitably) returned, they were left with very little acquired immunity and no malaria control program. Then came resistance: first, by 1969 fifty-six mosquito species had developed resistance to DDT; next, as a result of careless mass administration, drug-resistant malaria developed especially chloroquine resistance.

The MEP did have some successes. Malaria disappeared from 39 percent of the countries enrolled in the program. Parts of the Caribbean and eastern Europe became malaria-free. Still, in 1969, when it was clear the program was not working, the WHO shut it down. Intense focus on a single, technological solution to the malaria problem while ignoring the sociopolitical context of the disease; growing concerns over DDT's safety, especially after Rachel Carson's *Silent Spring*; pesticide and anti-malarial drug resistance; lack of financial commitment—all of these help to explain the failure of the MEP.

Since the 1960s malaria has made a startling comeback. In some places where there had been significant progress in malaria control, like India and Brazil, there has been a resurgence. At the beginning of the 1960s India had under a hundred thousand cases; by 1965 they had jumped 150 percent, largely due to ineffective monitoring and follow-up in states with less robust health infrastructures; unreliable sources of DDT, as well as resistance, contributed too. In Africa, where malaria had never been under control, things got worse. In Zambia and Swaziland malaria surged because of new agricultural developments, HIV/ AIDS, increasing poverty, and the eroding efficacy of pesticides and anti-malarial drugs. Increased population movements and a decrepit health infrastructure exacerbated the problem. Patterns of global economic development fostered growing economic inequality and massive debt, leaving fewer resources to combat malaria (and other diseases).

Malaria's resurgence has been met by another global approach to controlling the disease—the World Bank–sponsored Roll Back Malaria, begun in 1998. Roll Back Malaria, combined with the Global Fund for AIDS, Tuberculosis, and Malaria, has helped to draw attention to the disease, and this led to some increased funding. Yet malaria surges ahead. While not focused on eradication, and including Africa, Roll Back Malaria mirrors the MEP in some important ways. It has not taken into account what has been driving the resurgence in cases; it operated in places where the health infrastructure was weak; its efforts were not coordinated with other development work; and it has failed to take into account local conditions. While insecticide-treated bed nets, its key technology, have worked well in many places—the WHO claims they have been responsible for cutting malaria rates in half in Africa since 2000—they have also been repurposed, on a massive scale, as fishing nets in Nigeria, Mozambique, and elsewhere. Given the choice between fishing for food and using the nets for their intended purpose, millions are choosing food. The increase in fishing is having an adverse effect on fish stocks. A technology designed to help people stave off malaria is used instead to ward off hunger, but in the process the resultant overfishing is imperiling the very food source they rely on.

None of these programs focus on the conditions that give rise to malaria. The Gates Foundation directs much of its money to vaccine development; the foundation has also re-enlivened interest in eradication. And in May 2015, at the World Health Assembly, the WHO all but recommitted itself to eradicating malaria. A single-minded focus on one disease, however much the world would wish malaria gone, can have consequences. For example, although there has been success in reducing malaria in places like Zambia where it had been on the rise, it has recently been argued that this success has come at the expense of other types of health interventions. Focusing on a single disease like malaria can take resources away from programs that focus on general, overall health.

One of the greatest threats to malaria control is resistance. While resistance has been a concern since the advent of anti-malarials and insecticides, the problem has grown as it has been downplayed or more immediate problems held sway. Now artemisinin, long the most effective anti-malarial, is becoming less and less useful. At the beginning of the twenty-first century artemisinin resistance came to Cambodia; in early 2015 drug-resistant falciparum malaria had spread 1,500 miles—via human and vector migration—to the border between India and Myanmar. If artemisinin-resistant malaria spreads to Africa, the results will be catastrophic.

Finding a technological solution to the malaria problem, whether it be bed nets or more effective drugs, has been the dream of malaria control since the end of the nineteenth century; it is the central tenet at the heart of the gospel of control. The appeal is obvious. And by the middle of the twentieth century it seemed like all the pieces were in place to achieve what seemed the far easier goal of eliminating the vector via technology instead of eliminating, or mitigating, the conditions that help malaria flourish in the first place.

Chapter 4
Cholera

Cholera is a horrific disease acquired by ingesting water contaminated with infected fecal matter. Its symptoms—pallid, drawn skin; a gray and ghostlike appearance; rapid and often fatal evacuation of all bodily fluids—are shocking and appear quickly after infection with *Vibrio cholerae*. For centuries no one knew how to treat it. Then, in the 1960s, medical researchers and clinicians working in Bangladesh determined that a combination of salt, sugar, and water could replace the fluids lost to cholera (and diarrhea generally). Oral rehydration therapy has since saved millions of lives.

Though cholera had been present in India since at least the eighteenth century, the 1817 epidemic, because of its size and severity, is conventionally thought of as the beginning of cholera's history as a globetrotting pandemic disease. Since then seven cholera pandemics have traveled the globe. The first six were what is called "classical cholera" (*V. cholerae* O1). Each eventually petered out and cholera retreated to South Asia. For thirty-eight years, between 1923 and 1961, pandemic cholera disappeared. Then, for reasons still unknown, the El Tor biotype—named after its place of discovery in Egypt—began to replace classical cholera, and the ongoing seventh pandemic began.

Cholera, unlike tuberculosis, was not part of daily life; it appeared mysteriously, without warning, from the exotic and increasingly loathed and feared east. Its cause and cure were unknown. And as it became a disease of the urban poor and of immigrants from India and elsewhere, it came to symbolize filth and primitivism. Cholera exposed anxieties, revealed deep-seated divisions within medicine, and laid bare social and economic inequality in places such as Paris, London, Naples, and Hamburg.

While there are some themes in common—fear, debate over its causes and cures, horror over its symptoms and effects—each cholera pandemic has been different. The 1831–32 pandemic was far less severe in England than the 1848–49 pandemic—twice as many people died in the latter—but the public's reaction to it was far less panicked. The seventh pandemic—which we are in the midst of—has left Europe, where cholera has not appeared since 1911, unscathed. But it made its way in 2010 to Haiti, where it had not been seen for more than a century. Africa, which did not

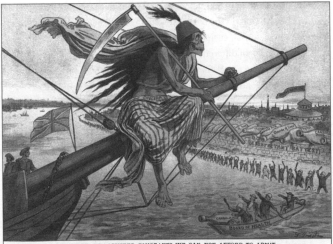

THE KIND OF "ASSISTED EMIGRANT" WE CAN NOT AFFORD TO ADMIT.

5. Fear of outsiders peaked during cholera epidemics. This 1883 cartoon shows an immigrant ship bearing cholera to America's shores.

confront severe cholera until the fourth pandemic in 1865–71, now suffers from more cholera than anywhere else.

The presence of cholera in one place and not another revealed to some observers essential differences between the clean and the modern, the filthy and premodern. A French writer, referring to what seemed to him to be a barbarian invasion from India, wrote in 1833, "There is reason to think that if the people of the banks of the Ganges had the good fortune to live under free governments they would tame the plague that their river is vomiting forth to poison other parts of the earth. The arm of liberty would snuff out the impure monster at its source."

Cholera symbolized a globe becoming smaller and more connected, its borders easily breached by the disease. The French delegate to the 1851 International Sanitary Conference noted:

Add now the communications between the peoples, today so numerous and more and more rapid; the navigation by steamship, the railways, and on top of that this happy tendency of the populations to visit each other, to mix, to merge, a tendency that seems to make of different peoples a sole and large family, and you will be forced to admit that for such a disease, so widespread and under these conditions, cordons and quarantines are not only powerless and useless, but they are, in the very great majority of cases, impossible.

Where did cholera come from? Beginning in the early 1830s, most thought the answer was India—Bengal, specifically—and Asia more broadly. Research into cholera's natural history in recent years has made its origins less certain—its protean nature, its clinical similarity to many other gastrointestinal ailments, its genomic instability, and its ability to flourish in marine environments worldwide suggest that the Asiatic cholera so confidently identified in the nineteenth century might not be exclusively Asian. This opens up the possibility that the cholera-like epidemics in Europe before 1817 were in fact cholera—a possibility shrugged off in the nineteenth century by those who could not imagine cholera having anything but an Indian origin.

The association of India with cholera has forever stigmatized that country. For reasons that are not entirely clear—perhaps this was a new strain; it might have been decades since cholera had broken out in India—the disease became especially virulent in 1817, leading to what a pair of East India Company physicians called, in 1819, "the most formidable and fatal diseases" to have "visited India in modern times." While estimates range, between 1817 and 1831 cholera likely killed millions of Indians, most of whom were poor and malnourished rural dwellers. Cholera spread across the entire continent, but Bengal was hit worst of all.

Cholera was more than a symbol of difference or of an interconnected globe. It was a physical presence. Its dramatic and sudden arrival in Europe in 1831 threw many into fits of fear; it signaled to some the arrival of a new plague. Some people fled, just as they had during plague epidemics; others stayed. Fear of cholera was at times out of proportion to the actual threat. In 1831, as cholera made its way through Russia, the anxious English awaited its arrival. Newspapers, pamphlets, and rumor spread fear of the disease. But Dr. James Johnson, editor of the *Medico-Chirurgical Review*, cautioned the press in a letter to *The Times*: "It will hardly be doubted that the terrible malady choleraphobia rages at this moment, epidemically, through every spot of the British Isles.... The choleraphobia will frighten to death a far greater number of Britons than the monster itself will ever destroy by his actual presence."

Seeing evidence of its destructive effects as it made its way across Russia toward Great Britain, a panicked writer warned in the *Quarterly Review*:

> We have witnessed in our days the birth of a new pestilence, which in the short space of fourteen years, has desolated the fairest

portions of the globe, and swept off at least fifty MILIONS of our race. It has mastered every variety of climate, surmounted every natural barrier, conquered every people. It has not, like the simoon, blasted life, and then passed away; the cholera, like the smallpox or the plague, takes root in the soil it has once possessed.

In Britain, in 1832, riots broke out in several locales. Coming on the heels of several well-publicized incidents of grave robbing, as well as one grisly and much talked about case of murder-for-corpse, the mobs directed their anger at doctors suspected of poisoning the poor in an effort to harvest bodies for medical school anatomy lessons. In France, some worried that the wealthy schemed to get rid of the poor with cholera. Cholera called into question the West's biological and cultural superiority: How could a disease from the primitive and backward East have the power to cripple the modern and progressive West? Cholera exposed horrific living conditions in the burgeoning metropolises of a rapidly industrializing Europe. Might it be that the very things making Europe modern were also those that caused cholera?

Misguided or not, fear matters. When cholera appeared in Naples in 1911, the Italian state so feared the potential consequences—reduced or halted trade and tourism; restrictions on emigration; the perception that Italy was not part of the modern, sanitary world—that news of the epidemic was hidden from the outside world.

Several of cholera's mysteries—mysteries it took most of the nineteenth century to answer and which were not limited to cholera—were especially important. Since not everyone suffered from it equally, many wondered why some got cholera and others did not. Was it contagious, as many by the 1830s believed smallpox and the plague to be? Did miasma cause it? Was it a combination of the two? To be a contagionist generally meant supporting such measures as quarantine. Those who believed in miasma thought quarantine useless; it was not people who transmitted the disease but the emanations of local effluvia—the rotting vegetable and animal matter in the soil and the bad air they produced. There was no strict divide between the two theories. Further, coming up with a sound theory was a challenge, because there was little methodological rationale for choosing some facts and not others; most tended to believe whatever suited their theory. A writer in *The Lancet* summed things up: "The progress of medicine, as an inductive science, is retarded by the construction of hypothetical theories, or the assumption of principles which are altogether gratuitous and imaginary, and also by the deduction of general principles or conclusions, from a limited number of facts."

While debates about cholera's route of transmission festered—and would for decades—something needed to be done in the short term. In this respect it seemed most were contagionists: from the liberal states like England and France to the autocratic ones such as Russia, Austria-Hungary, and Prussia, the initial response was to treat the disease based on historical experience with the plague and impose quarantine and restrictions on travel. States revived the practice of imposing a *cordon sanitaire* (sanitary border) in an attempt to keep cholera out; they kept careful tabs on the sick and the suspected sick, isolating them when possible; they blocked off infected zones; and they zealously disinfected, cleansed, and fumigated goods and people. As cholera approached Moscow in the fall of 1830, Russia mounted a vigorous defense—tearing up roads, destroying bridges, blocking passage into and out of the city. The military enforced restrictions on movement; disobedience meant death. Sixty thousand troops guarded two hundred miles of the eastern border. These severe measures were met with a mixture of indifference, fear, outrage, and resistance. Forced hospitalizations sparked popular unrest in Moscow and Saint Petersburg. In Vytegra, angry mobs freed patients held against their will; they destroyed hospitals.

The autocratic governments did not take a solely contagionist approach. They considered local conditions and instituted rudimentary sanitation measures—mostly toothless admonitions regarding hygiene—directed mostly at the poor. The possibility that cholera might have local causes, and the fact that it seemed to prey more upon the poor, suggested that the disease might not be just contagious. Growing ambivalence regarding cholera's method of transmission, popular displeasure at the severe restrictions placed upon daily life, and the merchant class's vehement opposition to quarantine and its effects on trade caused a shift to take place. As states, doctors, citizens, and public health officials gained more experience with the disease, the initial restrictions on trade and travel became increasingly difficult to enforce. Further, as evidence mounted that their effects were minimal, governments relaxed their approach. Additionally, as cholera traveled west along trade routes, the countries it entered drew on the experiences of those places that had already suffered—Russia, for example, had demonstrated that quarantine did not work. And thus, by the time the first wave of cholera in Europe was waning in the mid-1830s, belief in contagionism had waned. Fear of the disease, so strongly felt in the 1830s, never returned in the same degree. So different was the reaction to cholera when it came back in the 1840s and 1850s that places such as Lübeck and Hamburg in Germany adopted a policy of inaction; authorities worried more about the effects of trade restrictions and popular unrest than they did about cholera.

But once the initial shock of the first pandemic had worn off and the disease had retreated, reflection commenced. Relying on the historical experience with plague proved inadequate; alternative explanations and methods of control were necessary. The idea that it was strictly a contagious disease, passed from person to person, was cast aside. That it was a product of the local environment was not wholly satisfying either; not everyone in a given locale got it. Some believed that cholera was God's punishment for sloth and sin or brought on by its victims' immorality. Many began to notice an association between poverty and cholera. Living conditions might help to explain the disease's hold on some places and people.

The relationship between poverty and epidemic disease did not originate in the time of cholera; poverty and plague had long been linked. Yet in the 1820s and 1830s some began to probe the relationship in more detail. René Louis Villermé's demographic research in Paris in the 1820s established that one's economic standing, and not environmental factors, explained the ill health of the residents of Paris's poorest *arrondissements*. Villermé's British counterpart, William Farr, revealed similar connections in the urban centers of England. Cholera appeared as the result of poverty brought on by the rapid industrialization and urbanization spreading across much of the West. This way of thinking could comfortably accommodate contagion and miasma. It could be that the poor lived in miasmatic conditions, perfect for the spread of an infection like cholera. Environmental explanations for cholera came to dominate.

It was in England where this view went furthest in fostering public action. The association between a given place and cholera (and ill health generally) was most heartily embraced by Edwin Chadwick, who in the 1830s was a bureaucrat managing Britain's Poor Laws. Fascinated with the relationship between poverty and illness and committed to the utilitarianism of philosopher Jeremy Bentham, Chadwick teamed up with several physicians and in 1842 published the *Report on the Sanitary Condition of the Labouring Population of Great Britain*. Replete with maps, charts, and statistics demonstrating the correlation between illness, poverty, and the sanitary conditions of specific neighborhoods, Chadwick's *Report* became the bible of the British sanitary movement, which reached its apex in 1848 with the passage of the Public Health Act and the creation of the General Board of Health. Villermé thought that an unjust economic system created stark differences between the rich and the poor; Chadwick, a committed miasmatist, only saw dirty and clean places. There was no need for large-scale social and economic restructuring; cities simply needed to clean themselves up. Chadwick and his allies advocated a system of water delivery and sewage that would constantly flush out miasmatic waste. Chadwick's vision, which would take a half century to fully implement, would be, along with Paris's sewer system, one of the great engineering feats of the nineteenth century. And while clean water certainly resulted in healthier cities, concerns over the health of the poor were not always, or even often, the primary driver behind the clamor for clean water. Consumer and industrial interests demanded it.

To most who cared to look, the connection between urbanization, squalid living conditions, and disease was clear. People like Chadwick believed that clean water would flush away miasma and the effluvia of daily life that caused deleterious living conditions. That it might be the water itself did not occur to him. But it did occur to John Snow during his pioneering epidemiological work in London during the 1854 cholera epidemic. Snow had begun thinking about the problem of cholera during the 1848 epidemic, publishing *On the Mode of Communication of Cholera* in 1849. Snow wondered if the feces of cholera victims were infiltrating the water supply. To Snow, cholera, unlike smallpox, was not transmitted directly from person to person through the air, since it was a disease in the gut and not the lungs. That cholera was waterborne was just a theory—a theory he would soon be able to test.

In a legendary feat of epidemiology, Snow mapped the location of cholera cases during the 1854 epidemic to determine where those who got sick got their water. The connection became clear: in Soho, Snow revealed, those with cholera all drank water from the same source, the Broad Street pump. After Snow successfully lobbied to have the pump handle removed, cholera cases fell precipitously. It was clear: something was in the water. But no one yet knew what it was.

In the 1860s, as the balance of opinion began to sway toward believing cholera to be a contagious disease, there were still those for whom miasma was the best explanation. In India, some thought the subcontinent was so plagued by the disease because it was in the soil, traveled by air, and preyed upon a weak population uniquely susceptible to its ravages. The Indian sanitary commissioner thought quarantining ships or putting up a *cordon sanitaire* to keep cholera from traveling "would be no more logical or effectual than it would be to post a line of sentries to stop the monsoon." But this way of seeing cholera was at odds with where medical opinion was headed.

The death knell for miasma, though it did not ring loudly at first, was Robert Koch's bacteriological work in 1883, during the fifth cholera pandemic. After isolating the anthrax and tuberculosis bacilli, Koch set to work on cholera. When Koch discovered the comma-shaped cholera bacterium *Vibrio cholerae* in contaminated water and determined that it must be present to cause the disease, the end of miasma was in sight.

Koch's and Snow's work did not meet with universal approval. Miasma, often in attenuated form, still held sway. The influential German hygienist Max von Pettenkofer continued to argue for a clean water supply, not because he thought cholera was waterborne but because cleanliness in general was the key to good health. Cholera came from the emissions of contaminated groundwater as the soil decayed. For a time, Pettenkofer's views had a powerful effect on German sanitation policy, influencing, for example, Hamburg's decision regarding whether or not to provide clean drinking water to the city's poorest citizens (they did not). When cholera came to Hamburg in 1892 and not to neighboring Altona, where there was a clean supply of drinking water, those who believed in the waterborne theory of transmission—which by then included most medical scientists and others concerned with cholera—were vindicated. But Pettenkofer remained firm. To prove his theory, he drank water containing the cholera bacillus and developed diarrhea—but not, according to him, full blown cholera. As he saw it, the X factor (the bacillus) was not enough in the absence of the locally specific hygienic and climatic conditions (the Y factor) to produce a locally borne infection (the Z factor). But by the time of his experiment, views such as his were rapidly losing influence.

Contagionism took hold at the same time as sea and land travel were becoming ever faster, bringing the "civilized" West into increasingly frequent contact with the "uncivilized" East and its diseases. Concerns about the spread of the disease led to an era of neo-quarantinism, medical inspection, restrictions on travel, and a heightened form of medical internationalism. The International Sanitary Conferences, begun in the 1850s, were called regularly thereafter as a way for nations to come together and discuss the increase in global travel and trade. They became increasingly concerned with disease, especially cholera transmitted during the pilgrimage to Mecca, after the pandemic of 1865.

In previous pandemics it took half a dozen years for cholera to travel from India to Europe. In 1865 it took just two, as rail lines and steamship routes linked the Mediterranean with the Red Sea. By the 1870s the conferences had become a forum for discussing restrictions on travel from the Middle East and India. The Italian delegate declared in 1872: "We have to stop that cursed traveller who lives in India, everyone knows it, from taking his trips; at least we have to stop its progress as closely as possible to its departure point." It was not just India: the entire East posed a threat to the West. As a writer in the *Times of India* put it in 1892: "The actual danger for Europe lies in the international Mahomedan places of pilgrimage Mecca, Medina, Kerbalah, Damascus, Jerusalem, the different places in Persia and the large places of rendezvous of the processions of pilgrims.... Oriental squalor and the absence of any, or any serious sanitary police at the great places of pilgrimage encourage the disease whose germ finds a fertile soil in the bodies of the pilgrims, weakened by all kinds of deprivations." The "stranglehold on the east," as Mark Harrison called it, relaxed over time as countries like Italy and Great Britain began to balk at restrictions on trade and travel in an increasingly competitive global market that demanded the unrestricted flow of people and goods. At the same time, the association of the East, especially India, with cholera has never disappeared.

By the early twentieth century cholera had become more or less a thing of the past in western Europe and the United States. Italy suffered an epidemic in 1911, and the country's robust efforts to hide evidence of it make clear how rare and unwelcome it had become in rapidly modernizing Europe. By the 1920s, the disease had firmly lodged itself in the developing world, and the north lost interest.

The seventh pandemic has had the greatest effect in Africa—90 percent of cases. As Myron Echenberg rightly notes, the African experience forces a question: Why is it that at a time when we know more and more about cholera and possess a cheap and effective therapy has the disease only grown worse and claimed more lives? For the same reasons that TB and malaria continue to plague much of the continent, so too does cholera: since the 1970s, lack of health infrastructure, increasingly fragile economies, growing inequality, and poor sanitation all explain cholera's staying power. War-related population movements have aided cholera's spread.

The seventh pandemic in general has been quite different than the previous six. It is affecting new areas or areas not touched in a long time, like the former Soviet Union and Latin America; it has traveled very fast; it has lasted longer than any previous pandemic—it has been going strong for forty years and shows no sign of going anywhere; and El Tor is less virulent than classical cholera, which allows it to travel more easily.

Cholera, more than any other infectious disease, is the product and symbol of social inequality. It simply does not exist where there's a reliably clean supply of water. Climate change will likely make this worse as cholera's reach will expand into those places most affected by and unable to mitigate the effects of rising sea temperatures—temperatures at which cholera can thrive.

Chapter 5
Tuberculosis

Tuberculosis, caused by *Mycobacterium tuberculosis*, might be the oldest human disease. It is part of a family of mycobacterial diseases, including *M. africanum*, *M. bovis*, and *M. cannetti*, that have been evolving for perhaps three hundred million years. The oldest fossil evidence for a tuberculosis-like disease comes from a five-hundred-thousand-year-old *Homo erectus* skull found in Turkey with TB-like lesions. *M. tuberculosis*—the type that affects humans—emerged in Africa about seventy thousand years ago. It accompanied modern humans on their migratory paths out of Africa, first across the Indian Ocean and then, some millennia later, into Eurasia. TB flourished when people settled down and began living together about ten thousand years ago. It has been with us ever since.

Tuberculosis affects almost all parts of the body—the bones, the blood, the brain. Its most common and deadly form, carried in tiny droplets through the air from person to person and highly infectious, is pulmonary tuberculosis. It thrives in densely packed places.

Like plague, it is an ancient disease and has been written about for nearly as long. Tuberculosis was also discussed in terms of contagion and miasma. Retrospective diagnosis is tough. TB can look like pneumonia or other respiratory ailments. Centuries-old descriptions of its symptoms—night sweats, weight loss, hacking cough—make definitive diagnoses difficult. TB was the disease that ushered in the laboratory revolution, for it was the mycobacteria that causes the disease that Robert Koch discovered under his microscope in 1882. A disease once known as consumption and phthisis, with unknown but likely myriad causes, became a single disease—tuberculosis—caused by a single entity.

TB did not rise up and suddenly snuff the life out of millions like plague; it worked slowly. No one thought it the wrath of God, divinely sent to rout sin and sinners. Unlike cholera, its symptoms are not especially dramatic. One is not suddenly overwhelmed with TB, dead or alive in a matter of hours after disgorging one's bodily fluids. TB works insidiously, initially unseen. TB did not inflame the press and public like cholera did in the nineteenth century, nor did it arouse people to massacre others as plague did. Yet TB was responsible for far more death than either of these diseases. As early as the seventeenth century, the Bills of Mortality—the early epidemiological records from London—indicate that 20 percent of deaths in the city were due to consumption.

The ways people once understood TB were quite different than how it is now understood. Richard Morton's comprehensive *Phthisiologia*, published first in Latin and then in English at the end of the seventeenth century, considered consumption in all its many forms. For instance, to Morton TB could variously occur when people swallowed nails and punctured their lungs or when women expended too much breast milk and taxed their blood, leading to a weak, phlegmatic condition. While these do not sound like modern TB, when Morton talks about the tubercles, those knotty swellings in the lungs, his descriptions sound similar to the disease we now call tuberculosis. Thomas Sydenham thought long journeys on horseback were the soundest medicine.

Across the eighteenth century, descriptions of TB became more and more specific. Italian and British anatomists revealed tubercles in just about every part of the body. Vague descriptions began to disappear in the early nineteenth century after René Laennec unified all of the pathological descriptions of tubercle diseases then circulating. Without the tubercle, he wrote, there was no tuberculosis. Making his observations possible was the instrument he invented for listening to the body's interior, the stethoscope. Whereas previously a doctor would diagnose TB by listening to a patient's history and observing symptoms, Laennec homed in on the tubercle, revealing it with his stethoscope and after death with an autopsy. There was a clear path between Laennec's stethoscope and Koch's microscope. Beginning with Laennec and other Paris physicians who also focused on single-disease organisms, TB came into focus as a single disease. It gained a name, tuberculosis, in 1839 when the Swiss professor of medicine J. L. Schoenlein unified all the ailments for which there were tubercles under that title. Koch confirmed it all with his microscope in 1882.

Although it did not inspire the same kind of panic or xenophobia as did cholera, TB did become the subject of literature and opera (most famously Verdi's *La Bohème*) and the tuberculous romantic poet (Keats comes readily to mind) occupied a peculiar place for a time in nineteenth-century European culture. Upper-class female beauty in the form of a pale, wilting woman who rarely saw the sun, preferring to languish for long hours indoors, was not dissimilar to the consumptive: pale, thin, and weak. As TB assumed a more prominent place in European mortality, so too did it come to occupy a more prominent place in various aspects of culture. The romanticization of tuberculosis was but a small, and short-lived, feature of the disease's history, overshadowed by its enormous effects on the lives of those whom it affected most—the urban poor. Yet the images of the romantic poet wracked by TB or the wan woman prone on her daybed have had remarkable staying power.

TB took a larger place in the culture at large, and occupied the nineteenth century's most prominent medical minds, because it had firmly lodged itself in the body of the public. It was the nineteenth century's greatest killer. It increased apace with industrial development and the growth of crowded, unhealthy cities like Paris and London. Marx and Engels wrote in 1862 that "consumption and other lung diseases among the working people are the necessary conditions to the existence of capital." So inextricable were industrialization, urbanization, and TB that by the 1930s these were seen as necessary steps on a country's path to modernity. As TB increased in Africa and India just before World War II, it came to be called a disease of civilization. In the late 1930s, Lyle Cummins, a British TB expert and frequent commentator on the disease in the colonies, wrote that India was then where England was at the "time of the invention of 'Spinning Jenny.'" Charles Wilcocks, a British doctor with considerable experience in East Africa, echoed Marx and Engels when he wrote, nearly a century after them, of the increasing amount of TB in the burgeoning urban centers of East Africa, that "there is little care for human dignity in the life that breeds these conditions, and men become, not so much individuals as units of production." TB had become symbolic of the harsh conditions of modernity— modernity exemplified by a rapid increase in urbanization, industrialization, and the creation of a laboring class.

What happened in the developing world in the twentieth century happened in Europe in the nineteenth. Records are hard to come by, but it seems clear that TB was Europe's leading cause of death. In western Europe during the first half of the nineteenth century, mortality rates ranged from 300 to 500 per 100,000. By way of comparison, today in the United States that figure is about 0.1 per 100,000. TB began to take its industrial-scale toll first in England, where an epidemic of the disease ravaged the working-class population from the end of the eighteenth until the middle of the nineteenth century, by which time TB routinely claimed fifty thousand people per year in England and Wales out of a population of eighteen million. In its worst year, Cholera killed forty thousand.

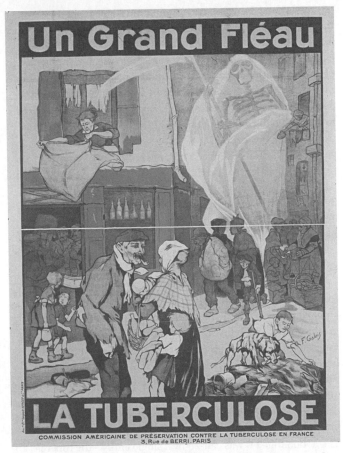

Un Grand Fléau

LA TUBERCULOSE

COMMISSION AMÉRICAINE DE PRÉSERVATION CONTRE LA TUBERCULOSE EN FRANCE
3, Rue de BERRI, PARIS

6. Slum conditions in European cities were conducive to the spread of tuberculosis. This 1917 poster shows a street scene from an impoverished area in Paris. The grim reaper is looming in the background.

While it is true that after about 1850 TB began a hundred-year decline, this does not mean the poor and working class were not still suffering from TB. They were, and disproportionately so. Once records began to be kept, they bore out what had been impressionistic. Postmortem examinations done in the 1880s at the London Hospital for Sick Children revealed that TB accounted for approximately 45 percent of mortality; 80 percent of these children were working-class. The same was true in Edinburgh: 39 percent of deaths at the Royal Hospital for Sick Children were due to TB; 98 percent of those children had been on public assistance. So great was the disease's impact in England that when it started to decline, so too did overall mortality. When one looks at France, Germany, Russia, or the United States, one sees similar patterns: growing industrialization accompanied by more and more TB. In the 1850s, in cities like Baltimore, Philadelphia, New Orleans, and Atlanta, TB was responsible for between 15 and 30 percent of all deaths. As it was across much of Europe, so too in America was TB the leading cause of death. Also like England and Wales, TB began to decline about mid-century. But the decline was uneven: it varied by location and social class; it also disproportionately affected racial minorities.

In the early spring of 1882, Robert Koch gave a talk in Berlin that stunned the world of medicine. He had identified the century's greatest killer, which he called the tubercle bacillus. The importance of Koch's work, its impact on medicine and public health, cannot be overstated. From then on TB had one single cause. Over time, the intense focus on the bacillus minimized, if not denied, the importance of the variety of social and economic causes of TB's prevalence among some populations and not others.

The notion that TB was caused by a single entity—the tubercle bacillus—did not catch on everywhere overnight, nor did it finally put to rest the debate between contagionists and anti-contagionists. Arthur Ransome, for one, was a prominent example of those who still clung to the view that diseases were not passed between people. Writing in 1887 in the *Transactions of the Epidemiological Society*, Ransome made what he considered a strong case for the soil being the agent. Though Ransome believed in the bacillus, to him, TB, like cholera, occurred in specific places;

it was not passed from one person to another. Ransome ascribed TB to fetid air: "It seems most probable, in fact, that for the active propagation of the disease, some increase in the virulence of the organism must take place outside the body, this intensification of its power being most commonly produced by the presence of animal organic matter in the air, in other words, by the absence of efficient ventilation. The favoring influence of a damp subsoil is also very distinct." However, by the early twentieth century most considered it contagious. In New York City, under health commissioner Herman Biggs, TB became an "infectious and communicable disease" in 1897, and a system of mandatory notification was put in place. Some states instituted compulsory hospitalization—a move some considered an assault on individual liberty for the public good.

The discovery of the cause of TB was cause for celebration—and overconfident predictions. The *Times* of London rejoiced at the likelihood that the "thousands of human lives which are now sacrificed every year to the diseases produced by the bacilli may at no distant period be protected against these formidable enemies." To great international fanfare, less than a decade after discovering the tubercle bacillus, Koch thought he had found a cure. But tuberculin, an extract of the tubercle bacillus that Koch hoped would act as a preventative, turned out to be useless as a cure (though quite effective as a diagnostic tool). Knowing the cause, it turned out, was only part of the solution to the problem.

Solutions to the TB problem included campaigns to outlaw spitting and attempts to build more adequate housing. One of the most popular and widespread treatments—and least effective— was sanatoriums. Part of the reasoning for the establishment of the first sanatorium, in the mountains of Silesia, was the belief that TB did not occur above certain altitudes. First appearing in Germany in 1859 and then popping up around northern Europe thereafter, the sanatorium craze came to the United States around the turn of the twentieth century. Designed to give patients a respite from busy city life and allow them to imbibe fresh country air, sanatoriums, it was hoped, would allow patients the time to heal. Absent an actual cure—no drugs and no vaccine existed yet—sanatoriums, in a way, harked back to a pre-Kochian view of the disease: they took people out of tuberculosis environments and put them into a healthy place.

Notions about altitude and TB changed, but the insistence on healthy outdoor living did not. In America, the cure for TB, advocated in such books as Lawrason Brown's 1916 *Rules for Recovery from Pulmonary Tuberculosis* and S. Adolphus Knopf's 1899 *Tuberculosis as a Disease of the Masses and How to Combat It*, was what came to be called the "outdoor life." Edward Trudeau most strenuously adopted the outdoor life at his sanatorium at Saranac Lake, New York, where patients braved the challenge of fierce winters by lounging outside in the hope that the fresh air would expunge TB from their lungs. Even though the relationship between cold fresh air and curing TB was unclear, even to its loudest boosters, Trudeau's sanatorium proved a great success: people came from far and wide to seek its cures. Philanthropy paid for the poor; the rich built their own cottages. Trudeau's sanatorium was private, but others were public. State or municipal governments, and in the case of American Indians the federal government, also ran sanatoriums. In the United Kingdom and much of western Europe, they were also run by the state. Many of them lacked the bucolic surroundings found at Saranac Lake, but they all emphasized rest, good diet, and plenty of time outside.

There were other attempts at a cure. The sanatorium treatment was essentially a passive affair; one mostly rested. Surgical solutions could not have been more different. The most common for pulmonary tuberculosis was collapse therapy, or artificial pneumothorax, which deflated the lung, allowing it to rest and heal. As Esmond Long, an American TB specialist, wrote in 1919, "The theory of artificial pneumothorax is simple enough.... [It is] the same as that back of bed rest or of lying, day in and day out, in a reclining 'cure chair,'—functional rest, enforced rest of the cured part [of the lung]." While Long was hesitant to go "too deeply into statistics," anecdotal evidence suggested it worked in what he called "desperate cases." The procedure surely had some positive effects in individual cases, but as a public health matter artificial pneumothorax was not a solution to the TB problem, nor were sanatoriums. Neither of these measures, as popular as they were, and as effective as they may have been in some cases, had any public health impact. Even when they were effective, they never served enough people.

TB demonstrably declined across the developed world, especially in the United States and Great Britain, between the middle of the nineteenth century and the era of antibiotics, thanks to specific public health measures and an improved standard of living. New public health departments in cities in the United States formed in part to combat tuberculosis. But no single cause can explain the overall reduction of TB in the general population. Segregating infectious cases in workhouses in Britain reduced TB in the general population by reducing the risk of infection. The same was true in New York: the identification and segregation of infectious cases by the newly formed public health department allowed for their removal from the general population to TB hospitals, thus reducing infection, and in this way sanatoriums had some effect. Reducing the risk of spreading infection was and is essential to stopping TB. But the resources necessary to do so have only been available in places where the standard of living has also increased. The absence of improved living conditions has been accompanied by an inability to reduce infections.

TB remained a disease of the poor. In New York, the large immigrant populations inhabited crowded, poorly ventilated buildings. TB rates there were far in excess of those in more well-off neighborhoods. In 1890, the Upper West Side of Manhattan had 49 cases per 100,000. In lower Manhattan, where vast numbers of immigrants lived, the rate was 776 per 100,000.

Between the wars, mortality for African American children under five was as much as 374 percent higher than for white children. Among African Americans in places like Baltimore, infections had not been reduced nor standards of living increased as they had for many sectors of the white population. Bureau of Indian Affairs prevalence surveys in the 1930s found that in the Southwest approximately 75 percent of the Native American population was infected. One hundred percent of Pimas over twenty tested positive. In Saskatchewan, 29 percent of all Indian deaths were from TB. Tuberculosis showed no signs of declining among marginalized populations in the US before antibiotics. But when Selman Waksman's lab discovered streptomycin in 1944 and ushered in the antibiotic era, it was as if a miracle had been performed: a formidable disease without a worthy foe had now met its killer. However, among the general population antibiotics killed off what was already dying.

As TB declined in the general population in the developed world, it increased elsewhere. Surveys in many places—among the Maoris in New Zealand and American Indians and First Nations in the United States and Canada, and in East Africa and South Africa—revealed alarmingly high TB rates. By World War II, it had become, according to health officials in Kenya, the colony's leading cause of death. Precise numbers were hard to come by, but the survey work, an increasing interest in collecting health data, and anecdotal evidence all made clear that TB was on the rise in much of Asia and Africa and among indigenous populations in the Americas.

For a time, a variety of racial explanations dominated the debate over why TB was increasing. Peoples in the less developed parts of the world—the "native races"—were virgin soil for TB; they were uniquely racially susceptible; or they had not become "tubercularized." Black South Africans, American Indians, and African Americans were most frequently the objects of this way of thinking. In India race-based explanations had little purchase, but evolutionary ideas concerning civilization did. In 1933, the public health commissioner of Bombay expressed a widespread belief about modernization, industrialization, and urbanization in India:

> Most western countries are said to have already passed through the epidemic stage...but it is difficult to state exactly at what stage the disease is now in India. Some hold that the peak has not yet been reached, that India is still in the early stages, and that the extent of tuberculinisation of the population is midway between that of the African races and the highly industrialised and urbanised European races. This view may or may not be correct but the fact is that the disease is rampant.

Racial ideas were powerful, but not irrefutable. At the end of the 1930s, as more and more data became available, they began to crumble. In Tanganyika, British TB expert Charles Wilcocks determined through an extensive X-ray survey that black Africans had in fact been resisting TB all along; healed lesions proved it. (Similar research among American Indians simultaneously showed the same thing.) Wilcocks knew that his finding was of more than "theoretical interest." His research would give "ground for the hope that adequate treatment can be made effective, and that the alteration in the conditions of life and education, which is the subject of all public health work, can help to control tuberculosis." As a result of work like Wilcocks's and generally changing ideas about race, by the end of World War II most TB workers had abandoned racial reasoning. TB was a disease of poverty. But while racial explanations may have been eradicated, TB had not been.

Before World War II little had been done to combat TB among the world's marginalized. But then, very quickly, several developments came together to inaugurate what was the most productive time in TB control the world had yet seen. The formation of postwar UN agencies like the World Health Organization (WHO) and UNICEF was part and parcel of the postwar impulse—an impulse sparked by a variety of motivations such as Cold War competition for hearts and minds, humanitarianism, and economic interest in new labor and consumer markets—to develop what came to be called the Third World. Combined with the recent discovery of antibiotics that actually cured TB and the positive results from the large-scale American Indian trial of the BCG vaccine (bacillus Calmette-Guérin—named for the two French biologists who developed it in 1908), the time was ripe to tackle TB in the developing world. In 1953 the WHO, referring to its planned mass BCG vaccine campaign, was prepared to launch what it called the "largest mass action the world has ever known against one single disease." By the end of the 1950s the sense that biomedical technology could finally solve the TB problem was palpable. As the WHO put it in 1958: "The possibilities for developing a tuberculosis control programme based on measures which, when applied in a public health programme, will prove effective, acceptable to the population, and not too expensive for use on a mass scale, are today, for the first time in history, really very great. The two main elements in this programme are vaccination and the use of the anti-tuberculosis drugs."

BCG made its way around the world into tens of millions of bodies, and antibiotics showed extraordinary promise. But the challenge was enormous. Hope mixed with despair in the world of TB control—despair over conflicting reports on BCG's efficacy and serious problems getting antibiotics to work as well in the real world as they had in trials. Testing BCG and antibiotics became the focus of much of the work of the WHO, UNICEF, and the British Medical Research Council (MRC), especially in India and Kenya. Vaccination held great promise because it would prevent TB; antibiotics offered a cure. But BCG's efficacy ranged considerably. Before the war, there was anecdotal evidence of its value from the French and Belgian colonies, where it had been used extensively. In 1946, results from a controlled trial seemed to demonstrate that it worked well among American Indians. Yet, as it spread around the globe, it was proving to be less than promising. Then, in 1979, the results of the largest trial to date appeared. BCG had 0 percent efficacy among 360,000 south Indian test subjects. Why its efficacy has ranged so widely has never been adequately explained. Differing strains of vaccine, exposure to environmental mycobacteria, high rates of infection, exposure to sunlight adversely affecting BCG—all these explanations and more have been offered. What kept BCG going for so many decades was the hope that it would work and the very powerful sense that no other preventative existed.

Antibiotics incontrovertibly worked. But they were frequently rolled out in places unable to effectively manage them; supplies ran low; some drug combinations were expensive, toxic, and/or difficult to administer. Facing these challenges, researchers from the WHO and the MRC developed cheaper drug regimens and demonstrated that self-administration in the home was possible. But all the energy, expertise, and breakthroughs could not combat what became in some places a serious, at times insurmountable, problem: drug resistance. In less than a decade, Kenya went from having no antibiotics at all to facing a nearly uncontrollable epidemic of drug-resistant TB by the mid-1960s. The same was true in other places where antibiotics existed in the absence of an effective management system. For decades, the WHO and others ignored the problem or downplayed its seriousness.

The postwar assault on TB joined the simultaneous push to eradicate malaria (unsuccessfully) and smallpox (successfully) as a narrowly conceived biomedical solution to disease control. For TB, this was never enough. Critiques of this approach, like the robust resistance movement against the mass BCG campaign in India in the 1950s, were very rarely taken seriously. In India and elsewhere, the notion that improving living standards was the key to lowering rates of TB was all well and good, but it was unrealistic, most in the development business thought. Many more agreed with American TB expert Walsh McDermott, who argued that because of advances in biomedicine, TB was a "disease

[that] can be decisively altered *without* having to await improvement in the social infrastructure."

By the mid-1970s, innovation and energy in global TB control had disappeared. TB was a neglected disease. But it had not gone away. And those still left working on TB, as well as those who continued to be at risk of contracting it, faced their biggest challenge yet: HIV/AIDS.

Because HIV weakens the immune system, it is the perfect companion for TB. It leaves those who are HIV-positive more susceptible to becoming infected with TB, and it is very effective at allowing a latent TB infection to fluoresce into an active one. In 1987 two researchers wrote that the "combination of both diseases could be at the root of a horrifying hecatomb [sacrifice or slaughter of many victims] in the years to come." So serious was the problem that in 1994 the WHO and the International Union against Tuberculosis and Lung Disease warned that the "combined epidemics of HIV and tuberculosis present a public health challenge unlike any other faced this century." Despite the early recognition of the relationship between the two diseases, very little was done during the first three decades of the HIV pandemic to stem the tide of HIV/TB. Renowned TB and HIV expert Anthony Harries, along with several colleagues, thundered in 2010 that the response to TB/HIV had been "timid, slow, and uncoordinated. If this situation had been a war...our efforts would have been ridiculed as half-hearted and ineffectual." Sub-Saharan Africa has been hit worst of all. Largely as a result of its deadly companion, TB went from a prevalence rate of 146 per 100,000 in 1990 to 345 per 100,000 in 2003. TB is now the number one killer of those with HIV/AIDS. For decades a combination of factors conspired to allow the co-pandemic to flourish: global indifference to TB by the end of the 1970s, the appearance of a new disease teaming up with an old one, the early neglect of HIV/AIDS in Africa, and continued incoherence and lack of leadership on global AIDS.

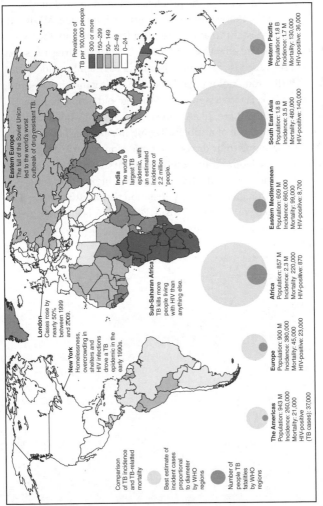

Prevalence of TB per 100,000 people
- 300 or more
- 150–299
- 50–149
- 25–49
- 0–24

Eastern Europe
The fall of the Soviet Union led to the world's worst outbreak of drug-resistant TB.

London
Cases rose by nearly 50% between 1999 and 2009.

New York
Homelessness, overcrowding in shelters and HIV infections drove a TB epidemic in the early 1990s.

India
The world's largest TB epidemic, with an estimated incidence of 2.2 million people.

Sub-Saharan Africa
TB kills more people living with HIV than anything else.

Comparison of TB incidence and TB-related mortality

Best estimate of incident cases proportional to diameter by WHO regions

Number of people TB fatalities by WHO regions

The Americas
Population: 943 M
Incidence: 260,000
Mortality: 21,000
HIV-positive (TB cases): 37,000

Europe
Population: 900 M
Incidence: 380,000
Mortality: 45,000
HIV-positive: 23,000

Africa
Population: 857 M
Incidence: 2.3 M
Mortality: 220,000
HIV-positive: 870

Eastern Mediterranean
Population: 609 M
Incidence: 660,000
Mortality: 99,000
HIV-positive: 8,700

South East Asia
Population: 1.8 B
Incidence: 3.5 M
Mortality: 480,000
HIV-positive: 140,000

Western Pacific
Population: 1.8 B
Incidence: 1.7 M
Mortality: 130,000
HIV-positive: 36,000

7. **Tuberculosis does not affect everyone equally. It is much more prevalent in some places than others.**

87

Added to the HIV/TB pandemic is the ever growing multi-drug-resistant (MDR) TB problem. Often billed as a new scourge, it is actually a continuation of the problem first encountered in places like Kenya in the 1950s and 1960s, only now it is worse. MDR-TB sufferers are resistant to at least isoniazid and rifampin, the two most common and effective antibiotics. Extensively drug-resistant (XDR) TB—which is resistant to isoniazid or rifampin and at least one of the fluoroquinolones and one of the injectable drugs—while new on its face, is also a new face of the age-old problem. Both MDR and XDR-TB are, like simple drug-resistant TB before them, a consequence of antibiotics being mismanaged at all levels: patients not taking their drugs; poor infection control; drug shortages; derelict program administration; the insistence, at times, that drug-resistant TB is simply not a big deal; and the more recent, though changing, perception that treating MDR-TB is not cost-effective. Like HIV/TB, MDR-TB has been neglected. Tuberculosis now kills more people than at any other time in history.

Chapter 6
Influenza

The influenza that swept across the globe in two waves in 1918 and a third in 1919 was the worst pandemic in history since the Black Death. Influenza had erupted into pandemic form before—most recently, and severely, in 1889–1892. But none approached the impact of the World War I era pandemic. It killed at least fifty million people. Most of that death came during the apocalyptic months of October and November. Looking back, the *British Medical Journal* wrote in April 1919 that in Bombay influenza "caused a havoc to which the Black Death…alone affords a parallel." It is still not known where the virus originated. Asia has often been cited. In Italy, rumors spread that it was not flu at all; it was chemical warfare perpetrated by the Germans. A pamphlet by an Italian doctor asked the question in its title: "Are the Latest Serious Epidemics of Criminal Origin?" The first known outbreak was at Camp Funston, Kansas, on March 5, 1918. From there it traveled to other forts and military facilities. It boarded ships bound for France in April. It spread quickly across Europe, reaching North Africa and India, and then going on to China and Australia by July. Flu struck so many longshoremen in the Philippines that dock work ground to a halt. The pandemic traveled the globe in four months.

The second, far more deadly, wave began in France in August 1918. It raced across the world via maritime trade and troop transport, appearing simultaneously in Boston; Brest, France; and Freetown, Sierra Leone. The Trans-Siberian Railroad carried it into northern Asia. Indian and British troops brought it to Iran, where it killed between 10 and 25 percent of the war- and famine-ravaged population. It arrived in Japan onboard a ship from the Siberian port city of Vladivostok, then under Japanese occupation. After it landed on the west coast of Africa, in Freetown—where the newspapers reported that the country "is all upside down…people are dying like rats.…the dead are now buried in trenches because of a lack of room in the cemeteries"—it made its way into the interior via newly opened rail lines. It came to Ghana without warning. A colonial official noted that in the north "Lorha is like a deserted village, one sees no one. I hear that some Lobis are wondering if this is the end of the world." Once it arrived in Cape Town, it quickly made its way north via railroad. Flu's spread across South Africa was swift, as the nation had one of the continent's busiest ports and the most well-developed internal transportation networks. It followed the Congo River aboard steamship almost back to the Atlantic Coast. Flu came to the other side of Africa via the Indian Ocean trade, first appearing in Mombasa in late September.

Within a few months the second wave had washed over nearly every inhabited place on the planet. The milder third wave arrived in the winter of 1919 and was gone by the spring. The pandemic was over.

The demographic effects were staggering. Half a billion people—a third of the world's population—were infected. Incomplete reporting and inaccurate diagnosis make coming up with a precise death toll impossible. In many of the places hardest hit, such as India and sub-Saharan Africa, demographic data were scanty, and the limited medical personnel kept few records. China, where the pandemic likely had devastating effects, did not begin keeping records until the 1930s. Given the virulence of the disease, actual mortality was certainly greater than the reported figures.

The numbers have changed substantially over the years. Edwin Oakes Jordan in *Epidemic Influenza: A Survey*, published by the American Medical Association in 1927, estimated the global total was 21.5 million. This remained the standard figure for decades, because so few had an interest in the pandemic. But historians have come to call Oakes's number "ludicrously low." As historians have taken more interest in the pandemic, they have revised Oakes's figures ever upward, sometimes significantly. While little is still known about places such as Russia and China, the most recent global estimate is fifty million; some think that figure may be an underestimate by as much as 100 percent.

Some countries, and even regions within countries, were hit much harder than others; mortality also differed based on age and gender. Indigenous people in Australia, New Zealand, and the United States suffered mortality rates as much as four times greater than the surrounding populations. In the remote native village of Wales in far northern Alaska, influenza was a virgin soil epidemic: 157 people died out of a total population of only 310. India, where approximately eighteen million died, had by far the highest death toll. Just as in other places, India's deaths from flu—mysteriously—were concentrated among young adults. This was quite different than previous flu epidemics and routine yearly outbreaks in which the elderly and the very young were disproportionally affected. In India women were hardest hit, because they took care of the sick. One result of both the age-specific mortality and the greater proportion of deaths among women was a marked lowering of the birth rate in India in subsequent years—as much as a 30 percent decline in 1919. There were fewer women, and many couples were no more.

The pandemic reached some of the most remote communities in the world. In the Pacific Islands the flu was devastating—mortality rates were higher in these islands than anywhere else. Almost no island lost less than 5 percent of its population. Western Samoa was the hardest hit: 22 percent of its population of about 38,000 died in a matter of weeks. If that happened today in the United States, seventy million would be dead. While the American naval administration was able to keep flu more or less out of American Samoa by strictly quarantining passengers on incoming ships and preventing mail boats from docking, such measures were never tried in Western Samoa. As a result, flu arrived aboard the New Zealand steamship *Talune*. Upon departure the ship had been given a clean bill of health, but in the week between its taking off from New Zealand and docking in Western Samoa flu became serious in New Zealand. No one warned Western Samoa or other ports of call. The islands learned about the pandemic from newspapers aboard the *Talune*, or from the devastating effects of the flu itself. Even though Western Samoa, like New Zealand, was part of the British Empire and the disease was well known all across the Pacific world, no one warned the islands of the unusually deadly nature of this particular flu outbreak. Within days, the island was overtaken. Ninety percent of the population was sick; social, administrative, and economic life ground to a halt.

The pandemic's virulence was blamed on the moral failings of Pacific islanders. The British agent on Tonga wrote: "The most discouraging feature of the outbreak was the apathy and indifference of the native chiefs to the suffering and distress of their people....When conditions were at their worst...not a single Tongan was procurable for the most urgent work." These moral failings had political consequences: "Such incidents cause one to revise one's estimate of the Tongan character and show them incapable of deep feeling and unfitted for the high responsibilities of self-government." The 95 percent morbidity rate left few capable of vigorous action. Yet British observers blamed the islanders for the lackluster response to the epidemic while cheering their own efforts as heroic.

So appalling was the death rate in Western Samoa and so many were the questions left in its wake—principally, how could this have happened in an increasingly well-connected world where news traveled fast?—that in the summer of 1919 the British Colonial Office formed the Samoan Epidemic Commission to investigate why influenza was allowed to pass to Western Samoa and other islands when it was successfully kept out of neighboring American Samoa. One of the questions was "whether the introduction and extension of the said epidemic was caused by any negligence or default on the part of any persons in the service of the Crown, whether in respect of the Executive Government of New Zealand or in respect of the administration of the said Islands of Western Samoa."

The answer was yes. The commission determined that administrative bungling caused the failure to relay any information on the flu. Further, the commission found, the British administration in Western Samoa did not take the epidemic seriously enough; doctors assumed that their command of modern medicine would prevent the worst ravages of the disease. The failure to communicate was not limited to Western Samoa. The Colonial Office notified no one; the colonies themselves did a better job of telling their neighbors if they had flu. The dissemination of news was haphazard at best. Since flu was not a notifiable disease, news reached a given colony only when, for instance, Sierra Leone and the Gambia chose to notify neighboring Nigeria or someone read about it in the newspaper, or, worst of all, when the flu itself appeared.

That the pandemic was devastating is clear. The reason why is anything but. Pandemic influenza was not new, nor would the 1918 event be the last. Pandemics have been a regular feature of human history since the sixteenth century. Flu has been a yearly visitor for much longer. There had been a pandemic just a generation before in 1889–1890, and there would be later ones in 1957, 1968, and 2009. There will likely be another. But the 1918 pandemic was different.

Influenza is a virus—one with three types, of which influenza A is the most lethal and widespread. It is a zoonosis—a disease transmitted to humans from animals. The 1918 strain had not been seen before; it took until 2005 to even identify the virus as a strain of H1N1 (where H stands for hemagglutinin and N for neuraminidase; both are proteins) that had several distinguishing features. It struck young adults at a rate twenty times higher than during previous flu pandemics and the regular seasonal outbreaks, which generally had (and have) a far greater impact on the young and the old. Infection often led quickly to a deadly form of pneumonia. Mortality was much higher than in any other flu pandemic. Three separate waves, stacked one atop the other, left no time to recover or prepare.

Why all this was so still remains largely a mystery, its severity especially so. What is known from archival samples of the virus— which in 2005 allowed for a complete genomic sequencing of at least the fall 1918 virus—is that it is the ancestor of all four of the human and swine strains of what are called H1N1 and H2N2 lineages. But when it arrived in 1918 it was novel. It is possible that it originated in humans and then jumped to pigs. Yet not enough is known to say for sure, nor is it clear when it split into its human and porcine lineages. The genetic similarities between modern swine and human flu as well as the long-term association between influenza in pigs and people led flu researchers to conclude that pigs were the likely intermediary between the constantly circulating influenzas in animals and periodic pandemics in humans.

Until 1997. That year a virulent, deadly strain of avian influenza from Hong Kong, known as H5N1, jumped to humans directly. But so far H5N1 has been transmitted only from poultry to humans; human-to-human transmission has not yet definitively happened. It has become clearer and clearer that influenza A's largest reservoir is in fact avian—waterfowl, specifically. The discovery that avian influenza can pass directly to humans has upended previous models of flu transmission and alarmed virologists—who once thought this impossible—and public health officials. Added to influenza's ability to jump from animals to humans and back is that it changes rapidly and often (this is why we need a new flu vaccine more or less every autumn) via a process known as antigenic drift. Reassortment is a form of antigenic drift that occurs when different strains of the virus are mixed to produce a new strain; this is what happened, it seems, in 1918, 1957, and 1968. In the future it is possible that H5N1 will change in such a way that it becomes transmissible between humans, causing a new pandemic in a population of susceptible hosts.

Because flu is such a shape shifter, a group of prominent influenza researchers wrote in 2010, "Despite continuing progress in many areas, including enhanced human and animal surveillance and large-scale viral genomic screening, we are probably no better able today to anticipate and prevent the emergence of pandemic influenza than 5 centuries ago, as shown by the completely unexpected emergence of the 2009 novel H1N1 pandemic virus."

While we know a tremendous amount about the disease, there is much that still eludes us. That elusiveness, combined with influenza's power, is humbling. The 1918 pandemic arrived at a time when modern medicine had a newfound confidence in its ability to discover the causes of diseases and then offer cures. Yet before the development of vaccines in the 1940s and beyond, it was utterly defenseless against influenza.

But medical science did not know that. Beginning in the 1890s influenza was thought, erroneously, to be a bacterial infection—called Pfeiffer's bacillus after its discoverer, the German infectious disease specialist Johann Friedrich Pfeiffer. During the pandemic a raft of vaccines appeared, as did countless attempted remedies. None worked. Bacteriology was of no use. It was not until virology had matured enough that influenza was determined, in 1933, to be a virus. During the pandemic nothing could prevent it or cure it.

In the colonies modern medicine was no more effective than the frequently criticized "native" medicine it was supposed to replace. Colonial officials and expatriate doctors registered displeasure with the ineffectiveness of Western medicine, which strengthened local peoples' ties to traditional healers. In Bombay, this led to renewed interest in Ayurvedic and Unani medicine. In Sierra Leone, colonial authorities' handling of the pandemic prompted an editorial in the *Sierra Leone Weekly News* to opine, "The epidemic ought...to be made a distinct point of departure in the history of our country. It has been made ten times plainer...that our welfare lies in our standing up and doing things for ourselves." Not actually having effective treatment did not stop doctors from offering a wide array of "cures." The native commissioner in Belingwe, Southern Rhodesia, achieved "remarkable results" from a combination of mustard plaster, castor oil, brandy, and what he called "pneumonia mixture." Others used paraffin and sugar. Confident at first in these remedies, colonial administrators and doctors eventually admitted that Africans saw these "cures" for what they were: quackery. The Native Department reluctantly admitted that the progress doctors and clinics had made in convincing people to abandon indigenous medicine vanished as people "lost much of their confidence in the efficacy of European medicine." Africans associated the taking of European medicine with death and sickness. In parts of Southern Rhodesia, Africans kept outbreaks of the flu secret, fearing that sufferers would be sent to the dreaded lazaretto (isolation hospital) or be forced to take medicine many considered worse than the disease. This is not to suggest that African responses were effective, or that abandoning European medicine for Ayurvedic helped. It did not. No system was effective.

When influenza first appeared in Bloemfontein, South Africa, initial reactions were muted. The city considered itself so healthy that a local guidebook called it "the South African sanatorium." So confident was the city in its ability to ward off ill health that in early October, while flu was killing people in west Africa, the local newspaper wondered how dangerous "our friend the ordinary common or garden influenza" could be. They soon had an answer as bodies piled up and hospitals became overwhelmed. An elder of the Dutch Reformed Church said later in October, "It seemed to me that it was the end of mankind." The shock thrust the municipality into action—cinemas and schools were closed; local pharmacists were compelled to make their "flu mixtures" available to the public at no charge; black South Africans were conscripted as laborers to dig graves.

England, a country with one of the most robust public health infrastructures, mounted one of the weakest responses. Armed with a newfound faith in germ theory, physicians were convinced that they could tackle the disease and refused to accept that they had no real preventative or curative measures. Further, many medical professionals believed that fear fostered flu's progress, causing people to run about spreading the disease. Public health officials urged calm. This, combined with their overconfidence in modern medicine, led them to downplay the severity of the pandemic. Publications like the *British Medical Journal* counseled silence and inaction: one editorial said, "When epidemics occur, deaths always happen. Would it not be better if a little more prudence were shown in publishing such reports instead of banking up as many dark clouds as possible to upset our breakfasts?" An editorial in the *Manchester Guardian* echoed this sentiment: "Terror is a big ally of the influenza, and if the public state of mind can be steered out of the channel of fright a long, long step will have been taken to conquer the epidemic." Overreaction was frowned upon, especially in the face of war. As the *Times* remarked in December: "Never since the Black Death has such a plague swept over the face of the world; never, perhaps, has a plague been more stoically accepted."

On the advice of doctors, London's Local Government Board did little more than order that cinemas be well ventilated. Because of the strength of their faith in the germ theory, which was capable of lulling people into thinking cures and preventions were imminent, insufficient resources were directed toward mitigating some of the flu's effects. World War I had a profound impact—on morale, on the availability of doctors (so many were away), on the availability of resources generally. It proved tough to mobilize Britain to fight both a war abroad and a pandemic at home. Arthur Newsholme, chief medical officer of the Local Government Board, wrote:

> There are national circumstances in which the major duty is to "carry on," even when risk to life and health is involved. This duty has arisen as regards influenza.... It has arisen among munition workers and other workers engaged in work of national importance.... In each of the cases cited some lives might have been saved, spread of infection diminished, some suffering avoided, if the known sick could have been isolated from the healthy; if rigid exclusion of known sick and drastic increase of floor space for each person could have been enforced in factories, workplaces, barracks and ships; if overcrowding could have been regardlessly prohibited. But it was necessary to "carry on."

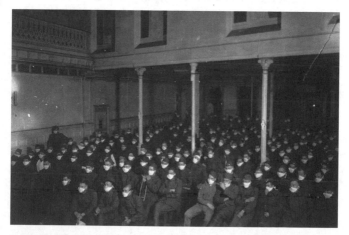

8. Fearing the flu, soldiers donned masks to watch a film in France during World War I.

Over the course of a few weeks in the fall of 1918, flu killed 250,000 people in England. Doctors and others distracted by war did not take the epidemic as seriously as they might have, but many people did recognize the magnitude of the crisis. As the *Times* put it: "So vast was the catastrophe and so ubiquitous its prevalence that our minds, surfeited with the horrors of war, refused to realize it. It came and went, a hurricane across the green fields of life, sweeping away our youth in hundreds of thousands and leaving behind it a toll of sickness and infirmity which will not be reckoned in this generation."

In the United States, initially, the Public Health Service published pamphlets that suggested the flu spreading across the country was in most ways no worse than the average annual flu. In the face of mounting cases, New York City's health commissioner continued throughout the first weeks of October 1918 to downplay the seriousness of the disease. Confident that the city could handle it, he cautioned citizens to remain calm; fear would only make things worse. In Italy, civil authorities forced the country's most influential newspaper, *Corriere della Sera*, to stop publishing the death toll as fear and anxiety mounted. These initially cavalier responses did give way to action in many places as municipalities realized the seriousness of the pandemic. Yet medicine was still ineffective.

Despite its failures, the appeal of modern medicine was scarcely diminished. The laboratory revolution had ushered in a new age; there was no turning back. Yet many physicians and public health experts were willing to admit their limitations. Thinking back on the pandemic in 1919, the bacteriologist Milton J. Rosenau wrote in the *Journal of the American Medical Association*, "If we have learned anything, it is that we are not quite sure what we know about the disease." This kind of admission was not uncommon, and at least in the United States it did not lead to despair; it pointed medical scientists toward opportunities.

The pandemic's effects are hard to gauge. Most historical work has focused on the pandemic itself, not what came after. Biomedical researchers, not historians, have taken the keenest interest. The appearance of H5N1 and the 2009 swine flu pandemic—which did not amount to the global nightmare that was predicted—sparked an extraordinary amount of research into the origins and implications of the 1918 pandemic. The pandemic has had a profound effect on twentieth- and twenty-first-century virology generally. But many historical questions remain. Some things do seem clear. For one, as a result of the disaster in the Pacific, as well as calls from New Zealand and South Africa to make flu a notifiable disease, there emerged a system of empire-wide disease surveillance and reporting. The system remained moribund until after World War II, but the pandemic did spawn an interest in a better system of international influenza surveillance—a system that is now considerably more robust.

But what of its cultural, economic, political, social, and demographic effects? From what little we do know, it seems to have had little impact in America. The pandemic has been all but forgotten. Its impact is barely detectable in memory or literature. Aside from the few books solely devoted to it, the pandemic rarely features in any substantial way in histories of the time. But could the same possibly be true in India, where nearly twenty million people died? Perhaps, but we don't know.

In many places in Africa—Southern Rhodesia, Nigeria, Zaire, and South Africa, for example—there arose a series of Pentecostal, or spirit, churches. The Aladura churches in Nigeria and the Kimbanguist Church in Zaire, for instance, formed when prophets, directed by God, appeared to save their people from the ravages of the flu. Pentecostal churches that emerged in Southern Rhodesia in the immediate aftermath of the flu's arrival remained long after the pandemic was gone.

In Bloemfontein, South Africa, the pandemic sparked a number of immediate changes in public health laws and invigorated a move toward poor relief as the city was forced to face the fact that it was not as healthy or as slum-free as it imagined. "The citizens were…shocked at the revelation of slums and degradation disclosed by the 'Flu'" announced the city's town clerk and treasurer. One of the city's newspapers, the *Friend*, wrote, "The immediate result has been a stimulating of the public conscience in the direction of long-delayed social reforms. Schemes are now under consideration which were regarded yesterday as the dreams of impracticable visionaries, and to-day are demanded as urgent necessities." Reform had been tossed about before, but it took the pandemic to shock the city into action. As the mayor told the Influenza Epidemic Commission, "Bloemfontein had long had such a scheme in contemplation, but the experience in the epidemic had hastened matters and stimulated public opinion, which was now ripe for these reforms." For now, one can only wonder if the pandemic caused similar reforms elsewhere, to say nothing of its possible effects on other aspects of life.

The 1918 influenza pandemic was an event. Unlike malaria and tuberculosis—the perpetual pandemics—influenza comes and goes. In this way it is more like smallpox or plague. Of course those two diseases are no longer major global threats. Influenza is. When H5N1 appeared in humans in 1997 and the novel strain of H1N1 turned up in 2009, the world was reminded of the possibility of another 1918. It has not happened yet. We do not know when it will. We are rather like the English in the seventeenth century. They knew that plague was out there, lurking, ready to strike, and they were more or less resigned to its return. They did not know when or why it would come back; they did, mostly, know how: by ship from abroad. Protecting themselves, once they knew it was coming, by keeping plague out was the only thing that had any potential of warding off an epidemic. We have vaccines now, a robust global monitoring system, and in some places a well-run public health infrastructure. Yet we are still like our seventeenth-century counterparts anxiously watching the shore.

Further, in the event of a deadly pandemic many of the same things that keep tuberculosis and malaria alive and well in the resource-poor parts of the world—among other things lack of public health infrastructure, inadequate access to preventive medicine, compromised immune systems, and rampant co-infections—will ensure that, just as in 1918, any future influenza pandemic will have wildly divergent effects.

While we are now sufficiently aware of the challenges of tackling the flu, and unlike in 1918 most virologists and public health officials do not possess an unhealthy amount of confidence, it can be hard to muster concern. For many, flu is simply synonymous with a cold. Both the 1976 swine flu and 2009's H1N1 pandemic amounted to much less than many public health officials predicted they would be. These things all can add up to a generally lackadaisical outlook when it comes to general concern about the possibility of a deadly pandemic. This is a mistake.

Chapter 7
HIV/AIDS

The arrival of HIV/AIDS was the end of the age of hubris. Any bluster about the death of infectious disease by the hand of biomedicine or hope of living in a world free of pestilence disappeared as it became clear that HIV/AIDS was a new infectious disease thriving in a world thought to be on the verge of being free of such menaces.

HIV/AIDS had been percolating in central Africa since the early twentieth century, but it appeared in its now recognizable form in the spring of 1981, when doctors in Los Angeles and New York City began noticing a strange uptick in rare diseases like pneumocystis carinii pneumonia (a fungal infection to which immunocompromised individuals are susceptible) and Kaposi's sarcoma (a rare form of cancer, mostly found in the aged). Even stranger was that they clustered in sexually active gay men. Then, over the next year or so, other groups, including hemophiliacs and intravenous drug users, became similarly afflicted. People from Haiti, too, seemed to be struck down. A Belgian doctor, Peter Piot, keeping up with the news from Centers for Disease Control, recognized similarities between what he was reading about in the United States and what he was seeing in his clinic in Antwerp—a clinic frequented by African immigrants. More and more reports from other parts of the world began popping up of unexplained cases of Kaposi's sarcoma and an assortment of immune disorders.

What linked these groups? Why were they all suffering from a host of diseases that were both rare and generally able to be fought off by a healthy immune system? The biomedical community snapped to attention. Initially (and unfortunately), the CDC labeled it GRID (gay-related immunodeficiency disease). In the summer of 1982 it was given its formal and lasting name: AIDS (acquired immune deficiency syndrome). Not long after, in 1983 and 1984, respectively, the Pasteur Institute in France and the National Cancer Institute in the United States identified the virus. Each called it something different; each claimed credit for the sole discovery. But soon the medical community settled on a name: human immunodeficiency virus.

HIV/AIDS has now killed nearly thirty million and infected nearly seventy-five million people worldwide. Tens of thousands of new cases appear each year. No part of the inhabited globe has been untouched by HIV/AIDS. But not everywhere is affected equally: well more than a third of all cases and deaths have occurred in southern Africa. In some places, like the Middle East, Latin America, Japan, and parts of Europe, HIV/AIDS affects mostly socially marginalized portions of the population; in central, eastern, and southern Africa it is a problem of the general population. In 2004, data from prenatal clinics in Swaziland revealed a prevalence rate of 42.6 percent.

When considered alongside the agents responsible for the causes of other diseases, the discovery of HIV only two years after AIDS first came to medical attention is remarkable—it took millennia to understand what caused plague. Decades of advances in molecular biology, immunology, and virology saw to that. The rapid identification of the virus and the seemingly limitless US federal government spending on medical research (the United States spent far more than any other country on AIDS research) led to hasty predictions of a vaccine and for a time bolstered modern medicine's confidence in its own powers.

But the optimism did not last. Identifying the virus was not enough. HIV turned out to be a complex retrovirus with several different identities. There are actually two viruses: HIV-1 and HIV-2. HIV-1 is more prevalent; HIV-2 is largely confined to West Africa and is much slower moving and harder to transmit. HIV-1 is broken down into groups (M, N, O) and then further into eleven genetically distinct subtypes (A–K). Group M (the main group) is the one responsible for the pandemic, as it causes 99 percent of cases. Subtypes A, C, and D make up the vast majority of cases, about 84 percent. Subtype C accounts for most cases in southern Africa, India, and China—and thus for a huge proportion of the world's HIV.

HIV 1 and 2 are both zoonoses (diseases originating in animals that now infect humans), and each of the different types of HIV is an instance of separate transmissions from chimpanzees (HIV-1) or sooty mangabeys (HIV-2). The greatest genetic diversity of HIV is in central Africa. All group M subtypes are found there, as are many recombinant forms in which the virus's genetic makeup is different still. Such genetic diversity means this is the region where HIV has been developing the longest and is thus the origin point for the pandemic. The virus passed from chimpanzee to human sometime around the turn of the twentieth century when, more than likely, infected chimpanzee blood entered the body of a hunter through a cut or open sore. By about 1920 HIV had made its way to the area around Léopoldville (since 1966 Kinshasa). From there it made its way across Africa along ever developing transportation networks. Its speed accelerated in various places and times: colonial era medical campaigns against sleeping sickness, yaws, and syphilis frequently reused needles, thus allowing the virus to be transmitted quickly to large numbers of people. Passing HIV to female prostitutes by treating them for syphilis with non-sterile needles was an especially effective way of getting HIV into the general population in the 1950s and 1960s. Once enough prostitutes were infected, HIV spread, especially in the dramatically changing environment of Léopoldville in the

1960s—mass migration to the city, high unemployment, and an explosion in prostitution. From there HIV moved on to Haiti as the many Haitians employed by various United Nations agencies like UNESCO migrated back and forth between the two countries. It then spread to the rest of the world.

HIV is very difficult to control. For one, because it is a lentivirus, it develops very slowly during a lengthy incubation. The genetic material of all life, including most viruses, is DNA. But HIV is a retrovirus, which means that HIV's genetic material is found in RNA (ribonucleic acid). When HIV invades a cell, it converts itself to DNA and then makes copies of its genetic material, via an enzyme called reverse transcriptase, as RNA. During the conversion, HIV makes many, many mistakes in copying itself, and the virus mutates. Because HIV changes so rapidly and so unpredictably, making a vaccine is difficult—so far it has proven impossible. HIV makes its way into the body via infected fluids—blood and semen are the most effective. Heterosexual transmission is most common. However, mother-to-child transmission, non-sterile needles used for intravenous drugs, and men having sex with men are all critically important routes by which the virus travels. Once in the body, HIV attacks the immune system's CD4 cells. Especially important is that HIV targets two types of CD4 cells essential for fighting infections: the T helper cells, which are the body's main defense against foreign bodies and infections, and the macrophages, which seize foreign bodies and allow the immune system to recognize these invaders. Once infected, seroconversion—the process by which HIV antibodies develop in the body and the virus becomes detectable—occurs. The strength of the infection is measured by viral load; a person is most infectious shortly after infection.

HIV progresses through four stages based on the CD4 count—a healthy individual's CD4 count is more than 1,000 cells per cubic millimeter of blood. At stage 1 the CD4 count is usually greater than 500, and the individual is asymptomatic. Once at stage 2

CD4 has dropped to between 350 and 499, and symptoms like weight loss and fungal infections may appear. In stage 3 CD4 count has dropped below 350. The individual is severely immunocompromised and susceptible to many opportunistic infections. Full-blown AIDS, when the CD4 count is below 200, is stage 4. As a virus, HIV's main features are its stunning complexity and insidious ability to disable the very system designed to repel it.

Added to all this are the political and social factors that determine its control. They involve sexual behavior, gender, poverty, and access to medicine, as well as political will—or lack thereof. Yet because HIV/AIDS arrived at a time of scientific triumphalism, a time when the biomedical community felt powerfully that a biomedical solution was best and was imminent, there has always been a tension between the social and medical aspects of dealing with pandemic. Very broadly speaking, the biomedical response has been nothing short of breathtaking. An entirely new scientific industry has been created. Breakthroughs in understanding were rapid and frequent. As a result, the disease went from a nearly always fatal, virtually untreatable affliction to a manageable chronic disease in less than a generation.

But the biomedical breakthroughs have not always been in sync with life outside the lab. HIV/AIDS is now treatable, but access to drugs is uneven, and new infections continue to demonstrate that prevention efforts have been only partly successful. From the very beginning of the pandemic the response has been fraught with many, many challenges. In the United States, for example, where the disease has primarily been associated with sexually active gay men and intravenous drug users, panic, fear, and moral opprobrium were common reactions. Conservative senators such as Jesse Helms blamed gay men: AIDS was retribution for sinful behavior. Needle exchange programs, which have a demonstrable public health benefit, have always been controversial, thought by many to promote illegal drug use. Many perceived government agencies like the Food and Drug Administration to be slow and ineffective at approving new drugs in a timely manner. As a result, a powerful and effective AIDS activist movement, exemplified by ACT UP, emerged to challenge bureaucratic dithering.

Safe-sex programs ran into opposition from those who considered abstinence the best way to avoid HIV/AIDS; condom use was also slow to take hold among men who visited prostitutes, and some men simply refused to use them at all; and as the epidemic began to level off in the United States, the use of condoms diminished. Outside the United States the national responses to the pandemic have been so varied that generalization is not possible. Some countries were passive, while others took a more active approach. Cuba instituted strict isolation of those who were HIV positive and mandated testing for the entire country. In Africa, Uganda confronted the epidemic head-on right from the start, advocating for and promoting a campaign aimed at reducing the number of sexual partners individuals had. Other countries, such as Zimbabwe, denied even having the disease within its borders.

If measured in dollars spent, papers published, careers launched, and breakthroughs achieved, the biomedical response to the pandemic was extraordinary. The political and social responses were less so. Writing in *The Lancet* in 2008, several prominent physicians from the pandemic's early years claimed that the global response "was for the most part delayed, grossly insufficient, fragmented, and inconsistent."

One area of striking neglect was Africa, which was both the origin point and the epicenter of the pandemic. The reasons are varied and complex and are both indigenous and endogenous. Most considered AIDS to be a gay disease, and thus considerable stigma was attached to it. There were exceptions: Uganda and Senegal publicly confronted AIDS, admitted it was present, and worked to confine their epidemics by not stigmatizing the ill. In South Africa, denialism reached a peak in the mid-1990s when President

Thabo Mbeki and his minister of health argued, following the American denialist Peter Duesberg, that HIV did not cause AIDS and thus newly emerging and effective drugs would be useless.

The WHO was slow to take notice. Four years into the pandemic, Halfdan Mahler, the director general, still did not consider HIV/AIDS a priority. He stated, "AIDS is not spreading like a bush fire in Africa. It is malaria and other diseases that are killing millions of children every day." Further, the pandemic looked much different in Africa. In the United States and much of Europe, where the vast majority of research was being conducted, the disease most affected gay men and intravenous drug users. Biomedical research and policy largely focused on the disease's profile in the countries where the research was taking place. Heterosexual transmission was initially rare and not considered a driver of the epidemic. Relief set in among some in the United States as it became clear that AIDS was largely confined to "high risk" groups; the tidal wave of heterosexual AIDS many feared never came.

The consequences for Africa were great. The dismissal of heterosexual transmission as unimportant in the United States meant that the burgeoning heterosexual pandemic erupting in Africa—so effectively documented by the pathbreaking work of Project SIDA in Congo—was initially ignored. This meant too that the burden of HIV in women went unexamined. By the time the WHO started its Special Programme on AIDS (soon renamed the Global Programme on AIDS; GPA) in 1987, the pandemic had been silently spreading more or less unabated.

Once the GPA was created and Jonathan Mann (who had been running Project SIDA in Congo and who would go on to become a legend in the HIV/AIDS world) hired to run it, global AIDS received unprecedented attention; donations to WHO skyrocketed. The GPA had success in working with Uganda and Thailand to dramatically reduce transmission, and Mann successfully turned to nongovernmental organizations for help. The GPA also made HIV/AIDS a human rights issue in an effort to reduce stigma and ensure that individuals would not suffer discrimination and persecution. For a short time, the WHO attempted to think of TB and HIV in unison, recognizing that HIV was having and would continue to have a considerable impact on TB. The GPA operated more or less autonomously— which led in part to its downfall—and was WHO's largest and best funded program. When Mahler and Mann addressed the UN General Assembly in the fall of 1987, it was the first time in history that a disease appeared on the assembly's agenda. WHO was the leader in tackling global AIDS.

But HIV/AIDS's time in the spotlight was short-lived. Mann resigned in 1990, after repeatedly clashing with the director general, Hiroshi Nakajima. The GPA lost momentum. Not long after, the WHO closed the GPA. AIDS work moved to a new agency, UNAIDS, in an effort to consolidate activities in one place. In the transitional years from the end of Mann's tenure to UNAIDS reaching operational capacity—albeit far below that of the GPA—global HIV/AIDS was left leaderless and adrift.

Not many people were paying attention anyway. So focused were they on the domestic epidemic that both the AIDS activist movement in the United States and the US government itself virtually ignored AIDS in the developing world. And, tragically, these were the very same years that the pandemic began to increase exponentially in Africa. While AIDS briefly occupied the global stage during the early years of the GPA, attention flagged, and by the early 1990s, even though the majority of cases were in the developing world, it only received 6 percent of global spending on HIV prevention. Due to profound neglect and craven political calculation much valuable ground was lost in the 1990s. When UNAIDS published its book-length history of the global response to the pandemic, it pulled no punches: during the decade and a half after the first case appeared, they wrote, "the world's leaders, in all sectors of society, had displayed a staggering indifference to the growing challenge of this new epidemic."

Beyond simple neglect, overall aid to developing countries declined dramatically in the 1980s and into the 1990s. UN agencies like the WHO suffered when donor nations like the United States during the Reagan years refused to pay dues (though for a time the GPA was an exception, as it received earmarked funds). Neoliberal economic policies forced countries to accept austerity in order to pay down their large burdens of debt. HIV/AIDS began to have an enormous effect on economies at the same time as the effects of structural adjustment programs continued to sap countries' already meager reserves just when they needed resources the most. The effects were staggering. One result, among others, was that funding for healthcare plummeted; many African countries introduced user fees—fees few patients were able to pay.

During these years, too, the World Bank gained in importance while the WHO declined. Beginning in 1987, the same year GPA opened, the bank began funding more and more health programs based on neoliberal principles which meant, among other things, that health interventions would be evaluated based on analysis of cost-effectiveness; it also meant that many countries' public health budgets sharply declined. As the bank took on a larger and larger role in funding health programs, it naturally gained more and more influence over what those programs looked like. One of the most powerful effects was coming to see disease interventions in terms of cost-effectiveness. This new way of prioritizing programs made its debut in the World Bank's 1993 *World Development Report: Investing in Health*, which signaled to the world, according to an editorial in *The Lancet*, that a shift had occurred "in leadership in international health from the World Health Organization to the World Bank." The bank sought to identify (and the WHO followed along) which diseases had the most deleterious effects on the economy—measured in what are called

DALYs (disability-adjusted life years)—while also being relatively inexpensive to treat. By any measure, according to those calculating things in such terms, treating AIDS was not cost-effective. Because the newly emerging class of antiretroviral drugs was expensive, they were not cost-effective in low income countries. Some HIV prevention efforts, such as condoms, were considered cost-effective, but they were very hard to implement.

Thus developing countries were in a strange, perhaps ironic, position: just as the holy grail of the global north's pursuit of a technological fix was in sight—highly active antiretroviral therapy (HAART)—the global south was told by the north it could not have it; it costs too much. It would be more cost-effective to work on preventing HIV instead. The very same economic imperatives that led the United States to fixate on a biomedical solution to the neglect of social interventions were now preventing an effective biomedical intervention from reaching those most in need.

The 1990s was a decade of neglect and lost opportunity. The global political response to HIV/AIDS in the 1990s was inadequate. The same cannot be said of biomedicine. In 1995 and 1996 two new classes of antiretroviral drugs had been discovered, tested, and released: the first were protease inhibitors—first saquinavir, and then the non-nucleoside reverse transcriptase inhibitors, beginning with nevirapine. At the eleventh International AIDS Conference in Vancouver researchers announced that when drugs from these two different classes were used in a triple combination, the virus could be suppressed and the patient's immune systems restored.

A disease that had been a death sentence was no longer fatal. One of these drugs, nevirapine, not only helped those with HIV; it could also prevent its transmission to babies. Mother-to-infant transmission had been (and still is) a challenging problem, but giving a dose of nevirapine to the mother just before birth and the baby just after has a dramatic effect on this route of transmission.

Where access has been greatest, mother-to-child transition rates have dropped significantly. Tragically, nevirapine was kept out of South Africa's antenatal clinics until 2002—when the Constitutional Court intervened to make them available—because of Thabo Mbeki's belief that HIV did not cause AIDS.

With the advent of these new drugs it was possible that AIDS could become a chronic manageable disease, thus altering the course of the pandemic. But they were expensive—prohibitively so for many people. They cost $10,000 to $15,000 per year and needed to be taken for life. Insuring access would be critical. Meanwhile, in the United States mortality from AIDS-related causes began dropping in the late 1990s—between 1996 and 1997 alone it fell 46 percent. The domestic epidemic became less urgent, and the international pandemic continued to be virtually ignored.

Added to this were arguments from some in global health leadership that treating AIDS in the developing world was neither cost-effective nor feasible for lack of infrastructure. Two articles in *The Lancet* made this claim. One claimed that "data on the cost-effectiveness of HIV prevention in sub-Saharan Africa and on highly active antiretroviral therapy indicate that prevention is at least 28 times more cost-effective than HAART." The other argued: "The most cost-effective interventions are for prevention of HIV/AIDS and treatment of tuberculosis, while HAART for adults, and home based care organized from health facilities, are the least cost-effective." Treatment and prevention were deemed mutually exclusive. In the world in which many operated, these kinds of stark choices were thought to be necessary. Further, the head of USAID told the US House of Representatives, Africans were generally incapable of taking such drugs even if they were available, because, among other reasons, Africans do not wear watches; their way of rendering time is different, and thus they would not be able to adhere to a treatment schedule.

But then a tectonic shift occurred. Beginning around the turn of the millennium there emerged a new way of seeing the pandemic. Global health became a priority for the United States government and major philanthropies such as the Bill and Melinda Gates Foundation. For example, in 2000 the United States funded antiretroviral therapy (ART) for no more than a few hundred patients around the world; by September 2009 the State Department claimed that the United States was providing ART for 2.5 million people.

What explains this shift in funding and interest? Drug policy and cost. For much of the 1990s second-line drugs for drug-resistant tuberculosis and ART were extraordinarily expensive. Many in global health accepted this as fixed costs rather than human constructions. In the early 1980s, ACT UP pioneered AIDS activism centered on access to treatment. In the late 1990s a new generation of activists emerged in South Africa and demanded access to antiretrovirals and answers to a series of hard questions: What does it mean to say the drugs cost too much? Who decides? Who sets prices? To activists the answer was that if high prices were set by people, then they could also be lowered. And if the cost of drugs dropped, then arguments about them not being cost-effective would disappear.

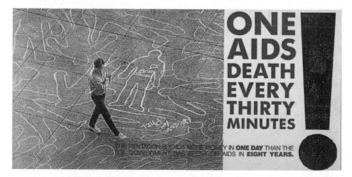

9. During the 1980s and 1990s, ACT UP drew attention to what many considered the lackluster US response to the AIDS epidemic.

Things began to happen on many fronts. Research began appearing to counter the claims of non-adherence and suggestions that prevention and treatment were mutually exclusive ends. Two studies of the limited role out of HAART appeared in 2001—one coming out of Haiti and the other out of Khayelitsha, outside Cape Town—that demonstrated people stayed on treatment. In the Cape Town study scientists learned even more: with the increase in availability of treatment, more and more people sought testing. That is, when people saw that there was effective treatment, more and more sought out AIDS services. As more people knew their status, and more began to receive treatment, transmission declined.

Clearly, HAART could work in resource-poor settings. But drugs still cost a tremendous amount. In India and Brazil, drug manufacturers began to produce cheaper generic versions of commercial ARVs. But in the rest of the world patents prevented drugs from being made in generic forms, and pharmaceutical companies, aided by the United States and the World Trade Organization, worked to keep generics out of global circulation. In 1997 South Africa attempted to challenge this by passing the Medicines Act, which stipulated that in the case of a public health emergency such as AIDS the country was allowed to both produce and import generic versions of drugs that were still patent-protected.

Claiming that the law violated their intellectual property rights, in 1998 thirty-nine drug companies reacted by filing suit in South African court. Activists, especially the Treatment Action Campaign, argued that the costs of the drugs were far out of proportion to their research and development outlay, to say nothing of the humanitarian argument for making them available.

The Clinton administration supported the drug makers, going so far as to put South Africa on a "watch list"—the precursor to sanctions—citing the possibility that the Medicines Act would "abrogate patent rights." When Vice President Al Gore announced

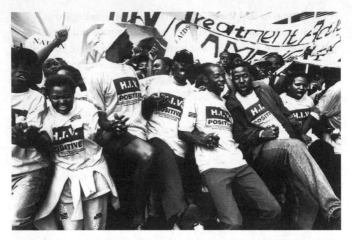

10. Treatment Action Campaign protestors demand free access to life-saving drugs in the streets of Durban, South Africa, in July 2000. This powerful image contradicts the popular perception of the disease and helpless "African" AIDS victims.

his candidacy for the presidency, protestors suddenly appeared behind him with banners that read "Gore's greed kills! AIDS drugs for Africa!" Protests broke out elsewhere, and within three months the US government reversed course: the United States would not pressure any country into purchasing only brand names and would allow importation of generics. By April 2001 all thirty-nine drug companies had dropped their suits. The door was now open for cheap generics to fill the gap in treatment.

Alongside the change in drug policy came a massive increase in funding. And one of the biggest funders—as well as one of the biggest surprises—was the President's Emergency Plan for AIDS Relief (PEPFAR), announced on January 28, 2003, during President George W. Bush's State of the Union Address. Bush said:

> AIDS can be prevented. Antiretroviral drugs can extend life many years.... Seldom has history offered a greater opportunity to do so

much for so many....To meet a severe and urgent crisis abroad, tonight I propose the Emergency Plan for AIDS Relief—a work of mercy beyond all current international efforts to help the people of Africa....I ask the Congress to commit $15 billion over the next five years, including nearly $10 billion in new money, to turn the tide against AIDS in the most afflicted nations of Africa and the Caribbean.

PEPFAR aimed to quickly scale up access to ARTs, modeled in part after work being done in Uganda.

By the middle of the first decade of the new century a combination of factors changed the face of AIDS funding and treatment: lower drug prices, growing evidence of the efficacy of treatment in resource-poor settings, grassroots activism, and new funding sources such as PEPFAR. However, access remains uneven, and new infections mean access will have to expand if the pandemic is to be stopped. Funding sources are fickle. Stigma and lack of understanding still hinder progress. Even in the United States, where activism and access has arguably been the greatest, African American men and women in places like Washington, DC, have rates far exceeding those of the white population—75 percent of new cases in 2013 were among the black population; likewise, 75 percent of those living with HIV/AIDS are black. During an outbreak of HIV among intravenous drug users in rural Indiana in 2015, it became clear that stigma was still a major problem when some addicts refused to get tested, as they feared being labeled as gay if they were seen coming and going from a local clinic; many did not know treatment was available or know the consequences of sharing used needles.

HIV/AIDS changed global health in fundamental ways: it spawned a vibrant and essential activist movement that changed the ways in which drugs are priced and accessed and also insisted on the link between health and human rights. The pandemic also made it clear that we will never live in a world free of disease.

It has also reminded us that we live in a world of starkly different opportunity and access—the fact that the overwhelming amount of HIV/AIDS is in the developing world should make this very clear. As with the other pandemic diseases, the global burden of HIV/AIDS rests on those least able to combat it.

Epilogue

What are we to do with this history? Does all this past experience, all this history, inform the present? Yes and no. In spring 2015 the WHO released a statement admitting its lackluster response to the Ebola pandemic and calling attention to a number of "lessons learned." It was a striking document. It was striking that in 2015 among the lessons learned were such things as the "lessons of community and culture." That it took Ebola to show the value of local people and their knowledge is surprising. The WHO "learned the importance of capacity"—which means the WHO learned that the world did not have the capacity to handle epidemics. The WHO was "reminded that market-based systems do not deliver commodities for neglected diseases." Why did it take Ebola to relearn that important fact? The WHO also learned that gains in such things as malaria control or women surviving childbirth can be reversed when "built on fragile health systems." Is it truly possible that this lesson had not been learned before 2015?

I am not interested in indicting the WHO—it is in this instance an easy target—and it is commendable that the leadership is admitting mistakes. But the WHO is, for better or worse, representative of a way of seeing things in the world of global health, and the leadership's statement on lessons learned allows me to make a point: every single lesson it learned (or in one instance relearned) could have been gleaned from a look at the past. These lessons are not new; the history of epidemics and pandemics has been teaching them for centuries. That there seems to be no historical consciousness is frustrating, but not just because I am a historian. It is frustrating because it is wasteful and inefficient. It is also arrogant and naive—a lethal combination. It is naive to think that by simply learning lessons the future will be different and arrogant to suppose that those proffering the mea culpas are the enlightened ones finally seeing the mistakes of the past. The WHO and others must ask: What are the origins of the mistakes themselves? That they were made is important, but the reason why might be more so.

Pandemics are not going away. There are no doubt more to come. A pandemic might come from an old and familiar foe such as influenza or might emerge from a new source—a zoonosis that has made its way into humans, perhaps. How will the world confront pandemics in the future? It is very likely that patterns established long ago will reemerge. But how will new challenges, like global climate change, affect future pandemics and our ability to respond? It is very likely that as the climate warms, disease-carrying mosquitoes, for example, will inhabit new places. Take the Zika virus. Carried by the *Aedes aegypti* mosquito—commonly referred to as the yellow fever mosquito—Zika exploded in early 2016 in Latin America and the Caribbean as temperatures set record highs and *Aedes aegypti* found suitable habitat. It is possible that as temperatures rise elsewhere, Zika will find a home further north. Rising water temperatures might provide more habitat for cholera. And as more and more research suggests a connection between the periodic rise in temperatures in central Asia and the arrival of plague in Europe in the late medieval period, we would do well to pay more attention to other instances of the historic connections between climate change and disease.

In the future, will nongovernmental organizations like Doctors Without Borders—the group that so heroically and tirelessly responded to Ebola while the world watched—be relied on as first responders? Or will the WHO regain some of its lost stature? One thing is clear: in the face of a serious pandemic much of the developing world's public health infrastructure will be woefully overburdened. One sure way to ease the suffering that will be encountered in any future pandemic is to invest in building a robust public health infrastructure anywhere one is lacking. The effects of pandemic and epidemic diseases have been and are going to be far worse in the places least able to respond. Although this might seem to be simple common sense, it is clear from the "lessons learned" by the WHO in the wake of the Ebola epidemic that it is still routinely forgotten.

References

Introduction

For the pandemic criteria see David M. Morens, Gregory K. Folkers, and Anthony S. Fauci, "What Is a Pandemic?," *Journal of Infectious Diseases* 200, no. 7 (2009): 1019–20.

Sanjoy Bhattacharya has written very effectively about the uses of history in contemporary discussions of epidemic disease: "International Health and the Limits of Its Global Influence: Bhutan and the Worldwide Smallpox Eradication Programme," *Medical History* 57, no. 4 (2013): 486.

Chapter 1: Plague

The quotes on the experience of the first plague pandemic are from Lester K. Little, "Life and Afterlife of the First Plague Pandemic," in *Plague and the End of Antiquity: The Pandemic of 541–570*, ed. Lester K. Little (Cambridge, UK: Cambridge University Press, 2007), 9.

For needing to employ such disciplines as zoology, archaeology, and molecular biology see Michael McCormick, "Rats, Communications, and Plague: Toward an Ecological History," *Journal of Interdisciplinary History* 34, no. 1 (2003): 25.

On the first plague pandemic in Britain see J. R. Maddicott, "Plague in Seventh Century England," *Past and Present* 156 (1997): 50.

The quotes from Ralph of Shrewsbury, the Paris masters, the *Decameron*, and the "French observer" are all from the essential volume *The Black Death*, trans. and ed. Rosemary Horrox (Manchester, UK: Manchester University Press, 1994), 112, 163, 26–27.

On Venice and Florence see Ann G. Carmichael, "Plague Legislation in the Italian Renaissance," *Bulletin of the History of Medicine* 57, no. 4 (1983): 511.

The details on labor shortages in England and Italy are from, respectively, John Hatcher, "England in the Aftermath of the Black Death," *Past and Present* 144 (1994): 3–35, and David Herlihy, *The Black Death and the Transformation of the West*, ed. Samuel K. Cohn, Jr. (Cambridge, MA: Harvard University Press, 1997); see 48–49 for Italian quotes. John de Wodhull is quoted in the manorial account of the royal manor of Drakelow in Cheshire, England, for 1349–1350. This is document 94 in Horrox, *Black Death*, quote on 283.

The Ibn al-Khatib quote is from John Aberth, *The First Horseman: Disease in Human History* (Upper Saddle River, NJ: Pearson, 2007).

Richard Leake and Stephen Bradwell are quoted in Paul Slack, *The Impact of Plague in Tudor and Stuart England* (Oxford: Clarendon, 1985), 39, 27.

The values quote is found in Vivian Nutton, "The Seeds of Disease: An Explanation of Contagion and Infection From the Greeks to the Renaissance," *Medical History* 27, no. 1 (1983): 31–32.

On earlier plagues not being *the* plague see Samuel K. Cohn, "The Black Death: End of a Paradigm," *American Historical Review* 107, no. 3 (2002): 737.

The president of the London Epidemiological Society is quoted in Mark Harrison, *Contagion: How Commerce Has Spread Disease* (New Haven, CT: Yale University Press, 2012), 185.

The *Mahratta* quote and the quote from the sanitary engineer are both in David Arnold, *Colonizing the Body: State Medicine and Epidemic Disease in Nineteenth-Century India* (Cambridge, UK: Cambridge University Press, 1993), 212, 232.

Chapter 2: Smallpox

The quote from Ho Chung is in Donald R. Hopkins, *The Greatest Killer: Smallpox in History* (Chicago: University Of Chicago Press, 2002), 104.

The quote from the Florentine Codex is found in John Mack Farther and Robert V. Hine, *The American West: A New Interpretive History* (New Haven, CT: Yale University Press, 2000), 22–23.

The quotes from the English colonists William Bradford and Thomas Hariot are from David S. Jones, *Rationalizing Epidemics: The Meanings and Uses of American Indian Mortality since 1600* (Cambridge, MA: Harvard University Press, 2004), 37, 26.

The concept of the Great Southeastern Smallpox Epidemic comes from Paul Kelton, *Epidemics and Enslavement: Biological Catastrophe in the Native Southeast, 1492–1715* (Lincoln: University of Nebraska Press, 2007).

For the Huron calling the French the "greatest sorcerers on earth" see Reuben Gold Thwaites, ed., *The Jesuit Relations: Travels and Explorations of the Jesuit Missionaries in New France, 1610–1791*, vol. 19, *Quebec and Hurons: 1640* (Cleveland: Burrows,, 1899), 91; this edition is a computerized transcription by Tomasz Mentrak, last updated April 14, 2011, available at http://puffin.creighton.edu/jesuit/relations/relations_19.html.

Truteau is quoted in Colin Calloway, *One Vast Winter Count: The Native American West before Lewis and Clark* (Lincoln: University of Nebraska Press, 2003), 419.

The Lewis and Clark quote is found in the online edition of *The Journals of Lewis and Clark Expedition*, based on the edition of the journals by Gary E. Moulton, available at http://lewisandclarkjournals.unl.edu/index.html.

Chapter 3: Malaria

The entomologist in Panama and *Mosquito Control in Panama* are quoted in Paul S. Sutter, "Nature's Agents or Agents of Empire?" *Isis* 98, no. 4 (2007): 743, 744.

Collins is quoted in Kenneth F. Kiple and Kriemhild Coneè Ornelas, "Race, War, and Tropical Medicine in the Eighteenth-Century Caribbean," in *Warm Climates and Western Medicine: The Emergence of Tropical Medicine, 1500–1900*, ed. David Arnold (Amsterdam: Rodopi, 1996), 73.

James Lind is quoted in E. C. Spary, "Health and Medicine in the Enlightenment," in *The Oxford Handbook of the History of Medicine*, ed. Mark Jackson (Oxford: Oxford University Press, 2011), 89.

Patrick Manson is quoted in Michael Worboys, "Germs, Malaria and the Invention of Mansonian Tropical Medicine: From 'Diseases in the Tropics' to 'Tropical Diseases,'" in Arnold, *Warm Climates and Western Medicine*, 194.

Bentley and Christophers are quoted in Ira Klein, "Malaria and Mortality in Bengal, 1840–1921," *Indian Economic and Social History Review* 9, no. 2 (1972): 142.

The Brazilian newspaper quote is in Randall M. Packard, *The Making of a Tropical Disease: A Short History of Malaria* (Baltimore: Johns Hopkins University Press, 2007), 96.

Paul Russell is quoted in Nancy Leys Stepan, *Eradication: Ridding the World of Diseases Forever?* (Ithaca, NY: Cornell University Press, 2011), 155.

McDermott is quoted in Walsh McDermott, "Environmental Factors Bearing on Medical Education in the Developing Countries," *Academic Medicine* 41, no. 9 (1966): S138.

The Cockburn quote is from T. Aidan Cockburn, "Eradication of Infectious Disease," *Science* 133, no. 3458 (April 7, 1961): 1058.

Chapter 4: Cholera

The Hamlin quote is in Christopher Hamlin, *Cholera: The Biography* (New York: Oxford University Press, 2009), 56.

For the quote from the French writer see Vijay Prashad, "Native Dirt/ Imperial Ordure: The Cholera of 1832 and the Morbid Resolutions of Modernity," *Journal of Historical Sociology* 7, no. 3 (1994): 247.

The quotes from the *Quarterly Review*, the *Medico-Chirurgical Review*, Durey, and *The Lancet* are all in Michael Durey, *The Return of the Plague: British Society and the Cholera, 1831–32* (Dublin: Gill & MacMillan, 1979), 7, 111, 111–12, 136.

The quote from the Indian Sanitary Commissioner is in Arnold, *Colonizing the Body*, 191.

The Italian delegate and the *Times of India* are quoted in Valeska Huber, "The Unification of the Globe by Disease? The International Sanitary Conferences on Cholera, 1851–1894," *Historical Journal* 49, no. 2 (2006): 464, 473.

Chapter 5: Tuberculosis

Marx and Engels are quoted in Helen Bynum, *Spitting Blood: The History of Tuberculosis* (Oxford: Oxford University Press, 2012), 112.

The Cummins quote is from S. Lyle Cummins, "Tuberculosis and the Empire," *British Journal of Tuberculosis* 31 (1937): 140–43, 141.

The Wilcocks quote is from Charles Wilcocks, "Presidential Address on Tuberculosis and Industry in Africa," *Royal Sanitary Institute* 73, no. 5 (1953): 481.

The Ransome quote is from Arthur J. Ransome, "Some Evidence Respecting Tubercular Infective Areas," *Transactions of the Epidemiological Society* 7 (1886–87): 124.

The Times quote is in David S. Barnes, "Historical Perspectives on the Etiology of Tuberculosis," *Microbes and Infection* 2, no. 4 (2000): 434.

The Long quote is in Esmond Long, "Artificial Pneumothorax in Tuberculosis," *American Journal of Nursing* 19, no. 4 (1919): 265, 268.

Public Health Commissioner of Bombay quoted in Niels Brimnes, "Languished Hopes" (unpublished manuscript in author's possession), 48.

The Wilcocks quote on lesions is in Charles Wilcocks, "Tuberculosis in the Natives of Tropical and Subtropical Regions," *Transactions of the Royal Society of Tropical Medicine and Hygiene*, 32, no. 6 (1939): 681.

The WHO quote on the largest mass action is in WHO, "Vaccination Against Tuberculosis, WHO Experts to Meet in Copenhagen," November 27, 1953, Press Release WHO/70, MOH 3/742, Kenya National Archives.

The WHO quote on possibilities is in Neil Brimnes, "Between Social, Cultural and Bacteriological Frames: Shifting Approaches to Tuberculosis in India c. 1920–1960," (unpublished manuscript in author's possession).

The McDermott quote on advances in biomedicine is in Walsh McDermott, "Tuberculosis at Home and Abroad," *Bulletin of the National Tuberculosis and Respiratory Disease Association* 54, no. 10 (1968): 11.

The Hecatomb quote is from J. Prignot and J. Sonnet, "AIDS, Tuberculosis, and Mycobacterioses," *Bulletin of the International Union against Tuberculosis and Lung Disease* 62, no. 4 (1987): 9.

The statement of the WHO and the International Union can be found in "HIV and Tuberculosis: Implications for TB Control Strategies and Agenda for Collaboration of AIDS and TB Programmes," WHO/TB/CARG(4)/94.4, Archives of the International Union Against Tuberculosis and Lung Disease, Paris, France.

The Harries quote is in Anthony D. Harries et al., "The HIV-Associated Tuberculosis Epidemic—When Will We Act?" *The Lancet* 375 (2010): 1906.

Chapter 6: Influenza

The *British Medical Journal* quote is found in Susan Kingsley Kent, *The Influenza Pandemic of 1918-1919: A Brief History with Documents* (Boston: Bedford/St. Martin's, 2013), 64.

The quote from the Italian doctor is in Eugenia Tognotti, "Scientific Triumphalism and Learning From Facts: Bacteriology and the 'Spanish Flu' Challenge of 1918," *Social History of Medicine* 16, no. 1 (2003): 101.

For Sierra Leone being "upside down" see Don C. Ohadike, "Diffusion and Physiological Responses to the Influenza Pandemic of 1918–19 in Nigeria," *Social Science and Medicine* 32, no. 12 (1991): 1395.

The colonial official remarking on the Lobis is in David K. Patterson, "The Influenza Epidemic of 1918–19 in the Gold Coast," *Journal of African History* 24, no. 4 (1983): 491.

On Oakes's figure being "ludicrously low" see Niall P. A. S. Johnson and Juergen Mueller, "Updating the Accounts: Global Mortality of the 1918–1920 'Spanish' Influenza Pandemic," *Bulletin of the History of Medicine* 76, no. 1 (2002): 108.

The quote from the British agent regarding Tonga is in Sandra M. Tomkins, "The Influenza Epidemic of 1918–19 in Western Samoa," *Journal of Pacific History* 27, no. 2 (1992): 190. The goals of the commission are in Samoan Epidemic Commission, *Samoan Epidemic Commission (Report of), Presented to Both Houses of the General Assembly by Command of His Excellency* (Wellington, New Zealand: Government Printer, 1919), 7.

The quote on how we're still unable to predict a pandemic is from David M. Morens, Jeffery K. Taubenberger, Gregory K. Folkers, and Anthony S. Fauci, "Pandemic Influenza's 500th Anniversary," *Clinical Infectious Diseases* 51, no. 12 (2010): 1444.

The quote on the pandemic being a "point of departure" is in Kent, *Influenza Pandemic of 1918–1919*, 111.

The quote from the native commissioner and the Native Department in Rhodesia are in Terence Ranger, "The Influenza Pandemic in Southern Rhodesia: A Crisis of Comprehension," in David Arnold, ed., *Imperial Medicine and Indigenous Societies* (Manchester, UK: Manchester University Press, 1988), 177, 178.

Quotes regarding Bloemfontein, South Africa, are in Howard Phillips, "The Local State and Public Health Reform in South Africa: Bloemfontein and the Consequences of the Spanish 'Flu Epidemic of 1918,'" *Journal of Southern African Studies* 13, no. 2 (1987): 211, 218, 224.

Quotes from the *British Medical Journal*, the *Manchester Guardian*, and Newsholme are in Sandra M. Tomkins, "The Failure of Expertise: Public Health Policy in Britain during the 1918–19 Influenza Epidemic," *Social History of Medicine* 5, no. 3 (1992): 440, 444.

The quote from *The Times* comparing influenza to the Black Death is in Niall P. A. S. Johnson, "The Overshadowed Killer: Influenza in Britain, 1918–19," in *The Spanish Influenza of 1918–19: New Perspectives*, ed. Howard Phillips and David Killingray (New York: Routledge, 2003), 155.

"So vast was the catastrophe" from the *Times* is quoted in David Killingray, "A New 'Imperial Disease': The Influenza Pandemic of 1918–9 and Its Impact on the British Empire," *Caribbean Quarterly* 49, no. 4 (2003): 32.

Rosenau is quoted in Nancy K. Bristow, *American Pandemic: The Lost Worlds of the 1918 Influenza Epidemic* (New York: Oxford University Press, 2012), 159.

Chapter 7: HIV/AIDS

For the slow global response see Michael H. Merson, Jeffrey O'Malley, David Serwadda, and Chantawipa Apisuk, "The History and Challenge of HIV Prevention," *The Lancet* 372, no. 9637 (2008): 475–88.

Mahler is quoted in John Iliffe, *The African AIDS Epidemic* (Athens: Ohio University Press, 2006), 68.

Project SIDA's work was documented in Thomas C. Quinn, Jonathan M. Mann, James W. Curran, and Peter Piot, "AIDS in Africa: An Epidemiologic Paradigm," *Science* 234 (1986): 955–63.

The UNAIDS quote is in Joint United Nations Programme on HIV/AIDS, *UNAIDS: The First Ten Years* (2008), UNAIDS/07.20E/JC1262E, 7.

On the shift from the WHO to the World Bank see "Editorial: The World Bank's Cure for Donor Fatigue," *The Lancet* 342, no. 8863 (1993): 63.

The two articles from *The Lancet* are Elliot Marseille, Paul B. Hofmann, and James G. Kahn, "HIV Prevention before HAART in Sub-Saharan Africa," *The Lancet* 359, no. 9320 (2002): 1851–1856, 1851, and Andrew Creese, Katherine Floyd, Anita Alban, and Lorna Guinness, "Cost-Effectiveness of HIV/AIDS Interventions in Africa: A Systematic Review of the Evidence," *The Lancet* 359, no. 9318 (2002): 1638.

South Africa abrogating "patent rights" is in Messac and Prabhu, "Redefining the Possible," 122.

For Bush's remarks see George W. Bush, "Address before a Joint Session of the Congress on the State of the Union, January 28, 2003," in *Weekly Compilation of Presidential Documents* 39, no. 5 (2003), available at http://www.gpo.gov/fdsys/pkg/WCPD-2003-02-03/pdf/WCPD-2003-02-03.pdf.

Further reading

General

The most comprehensive overview of epidemic and pandemic disease (disease in general, really) is Kenneth Kiple, ed., *The Cambridge World History of Human Disease* (Cambridge, UK: Cambridge University Press, 1993). William McNeill's *Plagues and Peoples* (New York: Anchor, 1998; originally published in 1976) is a classic. Particularly useful for writing this book have been Mark Harrison, *Disease and the Modern World: 1500 to the Present Day* (Oxford: Polity, 2004); J. N. Hays, *The Burdens of Disease: Epidemics and Human Response in Western History*, 2nd ed. (New Brunswick, NJ: Rutgers University Press, 2009); and Roy Porter, *The Greatest Benefit to Mankind: A Medical History of Humanity* (New York: Norton, 1997). An excellent collection of essays, including a superb introduction on what historians might learn from epidemics and why they are so fascinated with them, is Terence Ranger and Paul Slack, eds., *Epidemics and Ideas: Essays on the Historical Perception of Pestilence* (Cambridge, UK: Cambridge University Press, 1992). An excellent discussion of the ways in which we might think about epidemics and pandemics historically is Charles E. Rosenberg, "What Is an Epidemic? AIDS in Historical Perspective," *Daedalus* 118, no. 2 (1989): 1–17. For a guide to the literature on epidemics and pandemics generally see Christian W. McMillen, "Epidemic Diseases and Their Effects on History," *Oxford Bibliographies Online*.

Chapter 1: Plague

The literature on plague is enormous—larger than any other pandemic historiography. Much of that literature is focused on the Black Death. However, for an excellent introduction that covers all plague pandemics see Paul Slack, *Plague: A Very Short Introduction* (New York: Oxford University Press, 2012). Slack's volume in the Very Short Introduction series has an excellent suggested readings list that is more comprehensive than what follows. A classic, only available in French, is Jean-Noël Biraben, *Les Hommes et la Peste en France et Dans les Pays Europeens et Mediterraneens*, 2 vols. (Paris: Mouton, 1975).

For the first pandemic consult the essential Lester K. Little, ed., *Plague and the End of Antiquity: The Pandemic of 541–750* (Cambridge, UK: Cambridge University Press, 2007). Lawrence I. Conrad has studied the pandemic in the Middle East more thoroughly than anyone; see his "Epidemic Disease in Central Syria in the Late Sixth Century: Some New Insights from the Verse of Ḥassān ibn Thābit," *Byzantine and Greek Studies* 18, no. 1 (1994): 12–59, and "The Plague of Bilad al-Sham in Pre-Islamic Times," in *Proceedings of the Symposium on Bilad al-Sham during the Byzantine Period*, ed. Muhammad Adnan Bakhit (Amman: University of Jordan, 1996).

On the Black Death a worthwhile overview is John Kelly, *The Great Mortality: An Intimate History of the Black Death, the Most Devastating Plague of All Time* (New York: Harper, 2006). The most comprehensive history is Ole J. Benedictow, *The Black Death, 1346–1353: The Complete History* (Woodbridge, UK: Boydell, 2004). On the Middle East see Michael Dols, *The Black Death in the Middle East* (Princeton, NJ: Princeton University Press, 1977).

Beyond the Black Death there are many excellent histories. On the flourishing of medical writing on the plague see Samuel K. Cohn, *Cultures of Plague: Medical Thinking at the End of the Renaissance* (Oxford: Oxford University Press, 2010). The collection of essays edited by Vivian Nutton brings together many interdisciplinary perspectives on the plague: *Pestilential Complexities: Understanding Medieval Plague* (London: Wellcome Trust Centre for the History of Medicine, 2008). The plague's place in the Ottoman Empire is not as well understood as its role elsewhere. See Nukhet Varlik, *Plague and*

Empire in the Early Modern Mediterranean World: The Ottoman Experience, 1347–1600 (New York: Cambridge University Press, 2015), and Daniel Panzac, *La Peste dans l'Empire Ottoman, 1700–1850* (Louvain: Éditions Peeters, 1985). For the plague in early modern England see Paul Slack's indispensable *The Impact of Plague in Tudor and Stuart England* (London: Routledge & Kegan Paul, 1985). Carlo M. Cipolla's *Faith, Reason, and the Plague in Seventeenth Century Tuscany* (New York: Norton, 1979) is a model of historical writing.

The third pandemic has also benefited from much excellent historical writing. On the origins of the pandemic as it made its way through and out of China see Carol Benedict, *Bubonic Plague in Nineteenth-Century China* (Stanford, CA: Stanford University Press, 1996). For an overview of the pandemic in cities see Myron Echenberg, *Plague Ports: The Global Urban Impact of Bubonic Plague, 1894–1901* (New York: New York University Press, 2007). A good overview of the ways in which the global community tried to cope with plague, among other issues, is Mark Harrison, "Plague and the Global Economy," in his *Contagion: How Commerce Has Spread Disease* (New Haven, CT: Yale University Press, 2012), 174–210. The plague in India has been the subject of a number of excellent articles and chapters. See especially Rajnarayan Chandavarkar, "Plague Panic and Epidemic Politics in India, 1896–1914," in Ranger and Slack, *Epidemics and Ideas*, 203–40, and David Arnold, "Plague: Assault on the Body," in his *Colonizing the Body: State Medicine and Epidemic Disease in Nineteenth-Century India* (Berkeley: University of California Press, 1993), 200–239.

Chapter 2: Smallpox

Smallpox does not have nearly the same historiographical depth as the plague. There are, however, many excellent works that I have relied on. The only real overview is Donald R. Hopkins's *The Greatest Killer: Smallpox in History* (Chicago: University of Chicago Press, 2002). It is indispensable and covers the development of vaccination, for example, very well.

The literature on American Indians and disease generally is abundant. The debates over the population of the Americas in 1491 have gone on for decades. I have relied heavily on Elizabeth Fenn, *Pox Americana:*

The Great Smallpox Epidemic of 1775–82 (New York: Hill & Wang, 2001), and David S. Jones, *Rationalizing Epidemics: Meanings and Uses of American Indian Mortality since 1600* (Cambridge, MA: Harvard University Press, 2004). Paul Kelton has written two essential books that discuss smallpox: *Epidemics and Enslavement: Biological Catastrophe in the Native Southeast, 1492–1715* (Lincoln: University of Nebraska Press, 2007) and *Cherokee Medicine: An Indigenous Nation's Fight Against Smallpox, 1518–1824* (Norman: University of Oklahoma Press, 2015). James Daschuk's *Clearing the Plains: Disease, Politics, and the Loss of Aboriginal Life* (Regina, SK: University of Regina Press, 2013) does a superb job explaining how smallpox caused ethnogenesis on the Canadian plains and in the Great Lakes region. On bringing smallpox to the New World see Dauril Alden and Joseph C. Miller, "Out of Africa: The Slave Trade and the Transmission of Smallpox to Brazil, 1560–1831," *Journal of Interdisciplinary History* 18, no. 2 (1987): 195–224. Historians now generally reject the notion that American Indian susceptibility to disease was the sole cause of their demographic demise. Instead, they argue that population collapse was due to myriad factors such as warfare, competition over land, and malnutrition, among other things. See Catherine M. Cameron, Paul Kelton, and Alan C. Swedlund, eds., *Beyond Germs: Native Depopulation in the Americas* (Tucson: University of Arizona Press, 2015).

For vaccination's reception around the globe see the essays found in Sanjoy Bhattacharya and Niels Brimnes, eds., "Reassessing Smallpox Vaccination, 1789–1900," special issue, *Bulletin of the History of Medicine* 83, no. 1 (2009). Ann Jannetta's *The Vaccinators: Smallpox, Medical Knowledge, and the Opening of Japan* (Stanford, CA: Stanford University Press, 2007) and Brett L. Walker's "The Early Modern Japanese State and Ainu Vaccinations: Redefining the Body Politic 1799–1868," *Past and Present* 163 (1999): 121–60 are both excellent works on the connections between the history of state growth and infectious disease. For resisting smallpox vaccination see Nadja Durbach, "'They Might As Well Brand Us:' Working-Class Resistance to Compulsory Vaccination in Victorian England," *Social History of Medicine* 13, no. 1 (2000): 45–62. On this theme see Michael Willrich, *Pox: An American History* (New York: Penguin, 2011).

For smallpox in Europe see Hopkins, *Greatest Killer*, but also the chapters concerning smallpox in Peter Baldwin, *Contagion and the*

State in Europe, 1830–1930 (Cambridge, UK: Cambridge University Press, 1999). Also important is Ann. G. Carmichael and Arthur M Silverstein, "Smallpox in Europe before the Seventeenth Century: Virulent Killer or Benign Disease?" *Journal of the History of Medicine and Allied Sciences* 42, no. 2 (1987): 147–68.

William H. Schneider's overview "Smallpox in Africa during Colonial Rule," *Medical History* 53, no. 2 (2009): 193–277 is excellent.

The efforts to eradicate the disease are well covered in Sanjoy Bhattacharya, *Expunging Variola: The Control and Eradication of Smallpox in India, 1947–1977* (New Delhi: Orient Blackswan, 2006), and Nancy Leys Stepan, *Eradication: Ridding the World of Diseases Forever* (Ithaca, NY: Cornell University Press, 2011). The WHO chronicled its efforts in a massive and essential volume, now available electronically: Frank Fenner, Donald A. Henderson, Isao Arita, Zdeněk Ježek, and Ivan Danilovich Ladnyi, *Smallpox and Its Eradication* (Geneva: World Health Organization, 1988), available at http://apps.who.int/iris/bitstream/10665/39485/1/9241561106.pdf.

Chapter 3: Malaria

Randall Packard's *The Making of a Tropical Disease: A Short History of Malaria* (Baltimore: Johns Hopkins University Press, 2007) and James Webb's *Humanity's Burden: A Global History of Malaria* (New York: Cambridge University Press, 2009) are both essential reading, and I have based much of the chapter on these two books.

Malaria's arrival in and myriad effects on the New World is the subject of many books and articles. Among the best are Philip D. Curtin, "Disease Exchange Across the Tropical Atlantic," *History and Philosophy of the Life Sciences* 15, no. 3 (1993): 329–56; Mark Harrison, "'The Tender Frame of Man': Disease, Climate and Racial Difference in India and the West Indies, 1760–1860," *Bulletin of the History of Medicine* 70, no. 1 (1996): 69–93; and J. R. McNeill, *Mosquito Empires: Ecology and War in the Greater Caribbean, 1620–1914* (Cambridge, UK: Cambridge University Press, 2010).

On the ways in which malaria, migrant labor, and agriculture go hand in hand, see Alan Jeeves, "Migrant Workers and Epidemic Malaria on the South African Sugar Estates, 1906–1948," in Alan Jeeves and

Jonathan S. Crush, *White Farms, Black Labor: The State and Agrarian Change in Southern Africa, 1910–1950* (Pietermaritzburg, South Africa: University of Natal Press, 1997), 114–36. See also Randall M. Packard, "Maize, Cattle and Mosquitoes: The Political Economy of Malaria Epidemics in Colonial Swaziland," *Journal of African History* 25, no. 2 (1984): 189–212.

The effort to control malaria and the development of a variety of ways to do it is well told in Frank Snowden, *The Conquest of Malaria, Italy, 1900–1962* (New Haven, CT: Yale University Press, 2006), and Margaret Humphreys, *Malaria: Poverty, Race, and Public Health in the United States* (Baltimore: Johns Hopkins University Press, 2001). The difficulties associated with controlling malaria in Africa are the subject of James L. A. Webb, Jr., *The Long Struggle against Malaria in Tropical Africa* (Cambridge, UK: Cambridge University Press, 2014).

Nancy Leys Stepan's *Eradication: Ridding the World of Diseases Forever?* (Ithaca, NY: Cornell University Press, 2011) and Packard's *The Making of a Tropical Disease* are essential for understanding the impulse to eradicate generally and the Malaria Eradication Campaign specifically.

Chapter 4: Cholera

Two articles especially have had an enormous impact on the historiography of cholera and infectious disease generally. They are Asa Briggs, "Cholera and Society in the Nineteenth Century," *Past and Present* 19 (1961): 76–96, and Erwin H. Ackernecht, "Anticontagionism between 1821 and 1867," *Bulletin of the History of Medicine* 22 (1948): 562–93.

I have relied heavily on Christopher Hamlin's *Cholera: The Biography* (New York: Oxford University Press, 2009). It is wide-ranging and authoritative. Three excellent guides to cholera in Europe in the nineteenth century, especially the growth of the modern state and developments in medical theory, are Baldwin, *Contagion and the State*; Frank M. Snowden, *Naples in the Time of Cholera, 1884–1911* (Cambridge, UK: Cambridge University Press, 1995); and Richard J. Evans, *Death in Hamburg: Society and Politics in the Cholera Years, 1830–1910* (Oxford: Oxford University Press, 1987).

The growth of medical internationalism and cholera are best chronicled in William F. Bynum, "Policing Hearts of Darkness:

Aspects of the International Sanitary Conferences," *History and Philosophy of the Life Sciences* 15, no. 3 (1993): 421–34, and Valeska Huber, "The Unification of the Globe by Disease? The International Sanitary Conferences on Cholera, 1851–1894," *Historical Journal* 49, no. 2 (2006): 453–76.

Despite the overwrought title, Steven Johnson's *The Ghost Map: The Story of London's Most Terrifying Epidemic—and How It Changed Science, Cities, and the Modern World* (New York: Riverhead, 2006) is a compelling account of the work of John Snow and the changing ideas concerning disease transmission.

On cholera in India, David Arnold's *Colonizing the Body* is the place to start.

Myron Echenberg's *Africa in the Time of Cholera: A History of Pandemics from 1817 to the Present* (Cambridge, UK: Cambridge University Press, 2011) is essential. On the United States see Charles E. Rosenberg, *The Cholera Years: The United States in 1832, 1849, and 1866* (Chicago: University of Chicago Press, 1987; originally published in 1966).

Chapter 5: Tuberculosis

There are several overviews of TB. Helen Bynum's *Spitting Blood: A History of Tuberculosis* (Oxford: Oxford University Press, 2012) is the most recent and the one I turned to most frequently. Frank Ryan's *The Forgotten Plague: How the Battle against Tuberculosis Was Won—and Lost* (Boston: Little, Brown, 1994) and Thomas Dormandy's *The White Death: A History of Tuberculosis* (London: Hambledon, 1999) are also very valuable.

On TB's effect on medicine and society in a variety of different places I have relied on the following:

For England: Ann Hardy, *The Epidemic Streets: Infectious Disease and the Rise of Preventive Medicine, 1856–1900* (Oxford: Clarendon, 1993), and Linda Bryder, *Below the Magic Mountain: A Social History of Tuberculosis in Twentieth-Century Britain* (Oxford: Clarendon, 1988). For France: David S. Barnes, *The Making of a Social Disease: Tuberculosis in Nineteenth-Century France* (Berkeley: University of California Press, 1995). For the United States: Samuel K. Roberts, Jr.,

Infectious Fear: Politics, Disease, and the Health Effects of Segregation
(Chapel Hill: University of North Carolina Press, 2009); Mark
Caldwell, *The Last Crusade: The War on Consumption, 1862–1954*
(New York: Atheneum, 1988); and Sheila M. Rothman, *Living in the
Shadow of Death: Tuberculosis and the Social Experience of Illness in
American History* (New York: Basic Books, 1994). For South Africa:
Randall Packard, *White Plague, Black Labor: Tuberculosis and the
Political Economy of Health and Disease in South Africa* (Berkeley:
University of California Press, 1989).

For efforts to control TB internationally with antibiotics and the BCG
vaccine, as well as the TB/HIV pandemic and neoliberal thinking, see
my book *Discovering Tuberculosis: A Global History, 1900 to the
Present* (New Haven, CT: Yale University Press, 2015).

An excellent collection of essays on the contemporary TB pandemic is
Matthew Gandy and Alimuddin Zumla, eds., *Return of the White Plague:
Global Poverty and the "New" Tuberculosis* (London: Verso, 2003).

Chapter 6: Influenza

On influenza pandemics before 1918–1919 see K. David Patterson,
Pandemic Influenza, 1700–1900: A Study in Historical Methodology
(Totowa, NJ: Rowman & Littlefield, 1986).

The 1918–1919 pandemic has generated a lot of excellent historical
work. It has also spurred much biomedical work concerning the
origins of the pandemic as well as why it was so severe, among other
things. There are several overviews of the pandemic in the United
States; all are well worth reading: Alfred W. Crosby, *America's
Forgotten Pandemic: The Influenza of 1918*, 2nd ed. (Cambridge,
UK: Cambridge University Press, 1989), which covers regions
outside the United States as well; John M. Barry's *The Great
Influenza: The Epic Story of the Deadliest Plague in History* (New
York: Penguin, 2004) is especially well detailed and has much on
the history of virology; Nancy K. Bristol's *American Pandemic: The
Lost Worlds of the 1918 Influenza Epidemic* (New York: Oxford
University Press, 2012) does an excellent job chronicling what the
experience of influenza was like as well as discussing the hubris of
modern medicine.

The global pandemic, especially its effects in places like Samoa, Africa, Iran, India, and England, has also been the subject of superb histories. For an overview see the essays in Howard Phillips and David Killingray, eds., *The Spanish Influenza Pandemic of 1918–19: New Perspectives* (New York: Routledge, 2003). On India see I. D. Mills, "The 1918–1919 Influenza Pandemic: The Indian Experience," *Indian Economic and Social History Review* 23, no. 1 (1986): 1–40. For the pandemic's effects in Iran, Amir Afkhami's "Compromised Constitutions: The Iranian Experience with 1918 Influenza Pandemic," *Bulletin of the History of Medicine* 77, no. 2 (2003): 367–92 should be consulted. The pandemic had a devastating effect in the Pacific islands, especially in Western Samoa. Sandra Tomkins, "The Influenza Epidemic of 1918–19 in Western Samoa," *Journal of Pacific History* 27, no. 2 (1992): 181–97 tells the story in all its gruesome detail. The pandemic's wrath in Africa is the subject of a rich body of work; some is cited in the references. For a guide consult Matthew Heaton and Toyin Falola, "Global Explanations Versus Local Interpretations: The Historiography of the Influenza Pandemic of 1918–19 in Africa," *History in Africa* 33 (2006): 205–30.

The place of flu in American life, science, and public health policy is discussed in George Dehner, *Influenza: A Century of Science and Public Health Response* (Pittsburgh: University of Pittsburgh Press, 2012).

Mike Davis's *The Monster at our Door: The Global Threat of Avian Flu* (New York: Owl, 2005) is a good overview of the world's preparedness and the conditions that might give rise to a pandemic.

Among the most accessible articles in the biomedical literature are Jeffery K. Taubenberger, "The Origin and Virulence of the 1918 'Spanish' Influenza Virus," *Proceedings of the American Philosophical Society* 150, no. 1 (2006): 86–112, and J. K. Taubenberger, A. H. Reid, T. A. Janczewski, and T. G. Fanning, "Integrating Historical, Clinical and Molecular Genetic Data in Order to Explain the Origin and Virulence of the 1918 Spanish Influenza Virus," *Philosophical Transactions of the Royal Society of London* 356, no. 1416 (2001): 1829–39.

Chapter 7: HIV/AIDS

The AIDS literature is massive; not much of it is historical. For a general introduction to the disease Alan Whiteside's *HIV/AIDS: A Very*

Short Introduction is an excellent place to start. A solid historical overview can be found in Jonathan Engel, *The Epidemic: A Global History of AIDS* (New York: Smithsonian, 2006). To understand the pandemic in Africa see Helen Epstein, *The Invisible Cure: Africa, The West, and the Fight against AIDS* (New York: Farrar, Straus & Giroux, 2007), and John Iliffe, *The African AIDS Epidemic: A History* (Oxford: James Currey, 2006). While Jacques Pepin's *The Origins of AIDS* (Cambridge, UK: Cambridge University Press, 2011) is the best single volume explaining where AIDS likely came from and how it traveled.

The activist movement and the origins of citizen scientists—and much more—are the subject of Stephen Epstein, *Impure Science: AIDS, Activism, and the Politics of Knowledge* (Berkeley: University of California Press, 1996).

For a detailed look at how the United States and many countries in western Europe confronted AIDS, see Peter Baldwin, *Disease and Democracy: The Industrialized World Faces AIDS* (Berkeley: University of California Press, 2005).

The neglect of the pandemic can be found in Greg Behrman, *The Invisible People: How the U.S. Slept Through the Global AIDS Pandemic, the Greatest Humanitarian Catastrophe of Our Time* (New York: Free Press, 2004).

Paula A. Treichler's collection of essays *How to Have Theory in an Epidemic: Cultural Chronicles of AIDS* (Durham, NC: Duke University Press, 1999) is essential reading.

The role of neoliberalism and its transformation of the WHO, the World Bank, and AIDS policy is very important. To understand this relationship see Nitsan Chorev, *The World Health Organization Between North and South* (Ithaca, NY: Cornell University Press, 2012), and Luke Messac and Krishna Prabhu, "Redefining the Possible: The Global AIDS Response," in *Reimagining Global Health: An Introduction*, ed. Paul Farmer, Jim Yong Kim, Arthur Kleinman, and Mathew Basilico (Berkeley: University of California Press, 2013),

111–32. This essay also covers the changes in thinking regarding access to drugs and their costs as well as AIDS activism.

For the myriad ways in which AIDS has changed global health see Allan M. Brandt, "How AIDS Invented Global Health," *New England Journal of Medicine* 368, no. 23 (2013): 2149–52.

Index

Note: Page references in *italic* refer to illustrations.